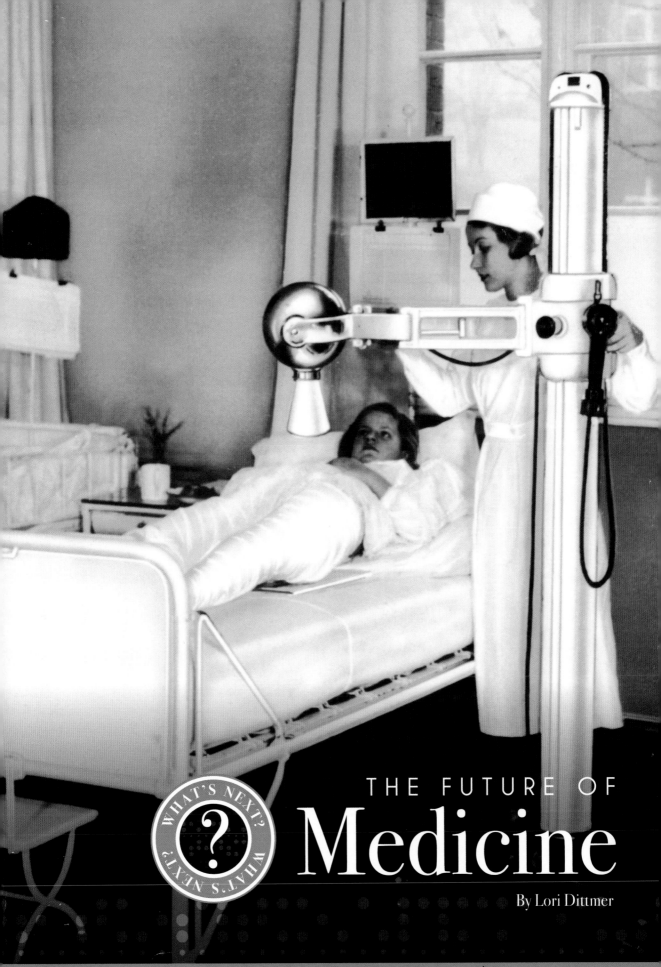

# THE FUTURE OF
# Medicine

By Lori Dittmer

CREATIVE ✦ EDUCATION

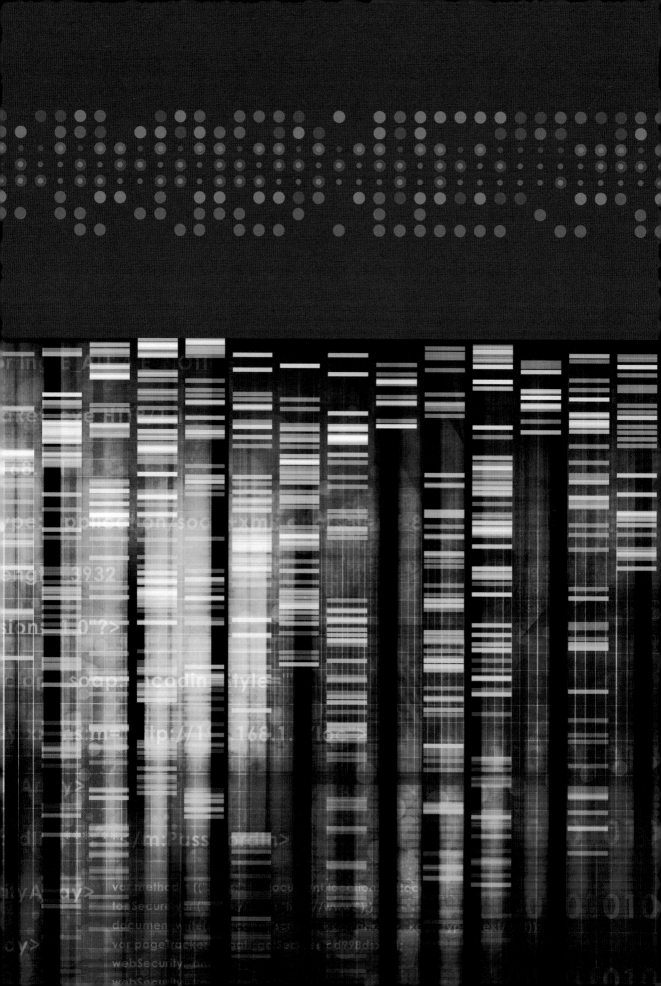

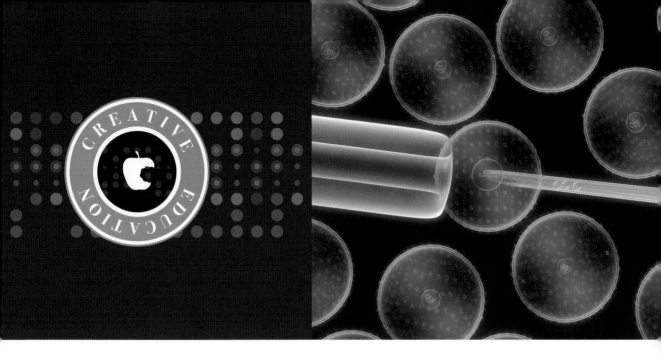

# TABLE OF
# Contents

# INTRODUCTION

What if you could get a medical checkup without visiting a clinic? Imagine simply touching your finger to a small device that draws a tiny amount of blood and promptly runs 2,000 different tests. The device sends the results to a computer, which sorts through a vast amount of information about your blood, organs, **genes**, and the way in which the environment is affecting your body. The results are e-mailed to you and your doctor. Checkup complete. Next, the doctor looks at the data from your blood to see whether you are at risk for certain health problems. Then, he or she might prescribe medicine to help prevent these conditions from developing.

Such a medical checkup seems far-fetched today, but as technology improves, we might indeed be able to undergo exams that are that quick and thorough. Throughout history, doctors and scientists have steadily improved medical treatments, from killing germs and developing disease-fighting drugs to performing life-saving surgery. A century ago, most people probably would not have believed that doctors would ever be able to transplant organs such as kidneys, hearts, and livers from one person to another. But the knowledge necessary for these surgeries accumulated quickly during the 20th century, suggesting the likelihood of more great leaps in the next century. Although we'll have to settle for traditional office visits for a while, a future of personalized medicine—in which a patient receives treatment according to the data provided by his or her own blood—awaits.

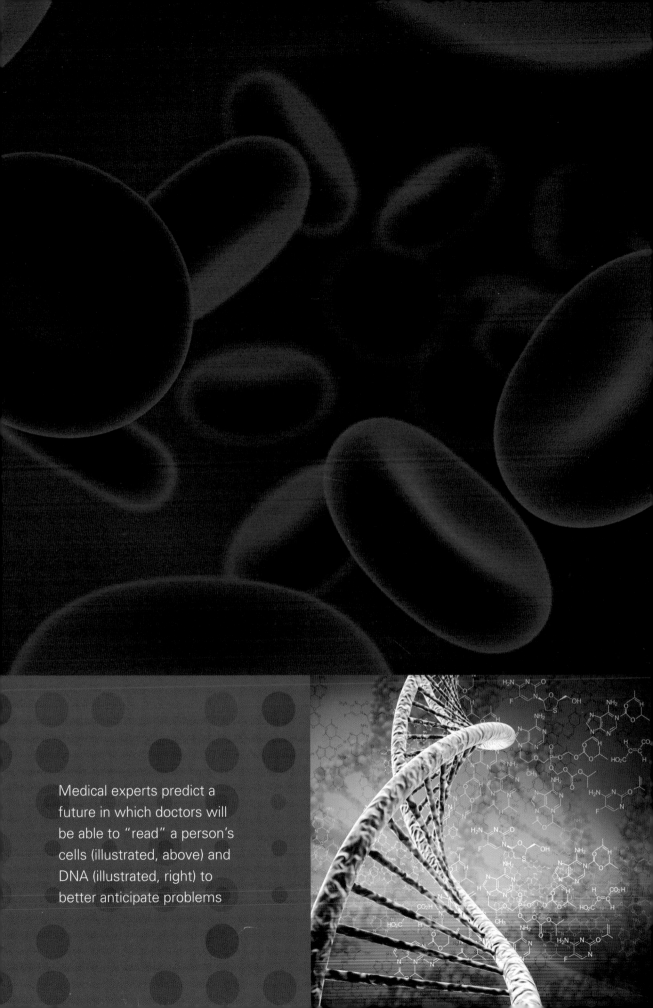

Medical experts predict a future in which doctors will be able to "read" a person's cells (illustrated, above) and DNA (illustrated, right) to better anticipate problems

CHAPTER ONE · CHAPTER ONE

# DISCOVERING GERMS, DEVELOPING DRUGS

**M**edical treatment among the earliest civilizations often involved sorcery and the supernatural. People blamed evil spirits for causing disease. **Archaeologists** have found ancient skulls showing evidence of trepanation, a procedure in which holes are drilled into a living person's skull. Although this surgery has been used in more modern times to relieve pressure from internal bleeding inside the skull, researchers believe that early doctors performed trepanation to release evil spirits from patients suffering from headaches or seizures, or those exhibiting bizarre behavior. In India, surgeons sometimes concluded operations with the help of large Bengali ants. After surgery, the doctor would place the ants next to each other at the site of an **incision**. After the insects clamped their powerful jaws down on the patient's skin, the doctor cut away the ant bodies, leaving the heads as stitches that eventually dissolved.

Ancient societies also used plants to treat illnesses. Medicine men who used these plants probably didn't know why certain plants helped specific ailments but could observe how people felt after eating the plants. Opium and black cohosh were found to ease pain, while figs were effective **laxatives**. Aloe helps to soothe skin conditions, and pomegranate kills **parasitic** worms in the intestines. These plants contain powerful healing substances, and many of today's drugs still include their ingredients. Ancient Egyptians were particularly skilled at using plants for healing sickness. In fact, the

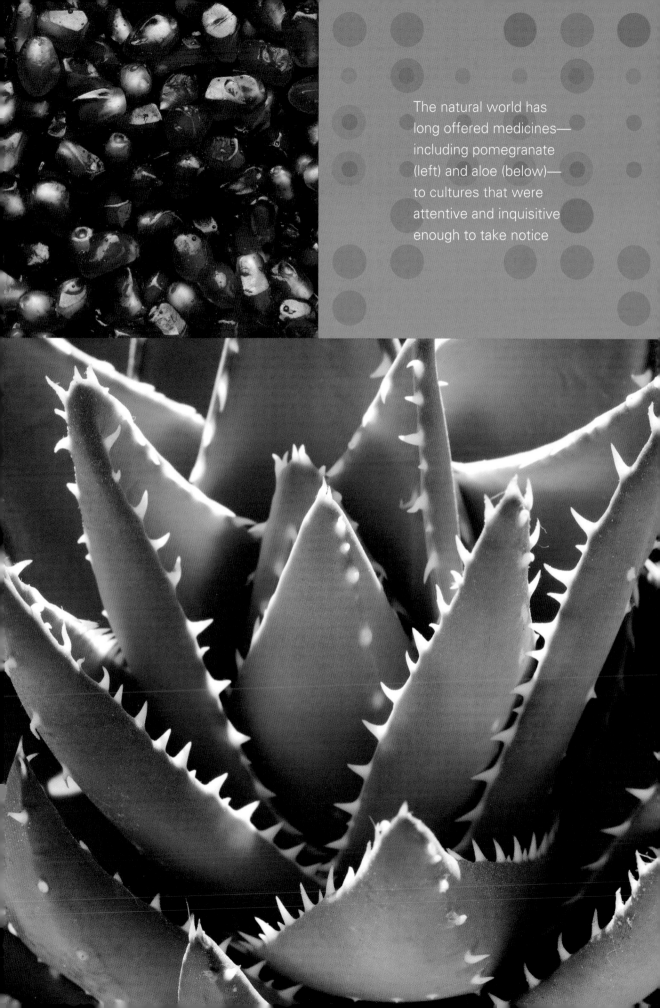

The natural world has long offered medicines—including pomegranate (left) and aloe (below)—to cultures that were attentive and inquisitive enough to take notice

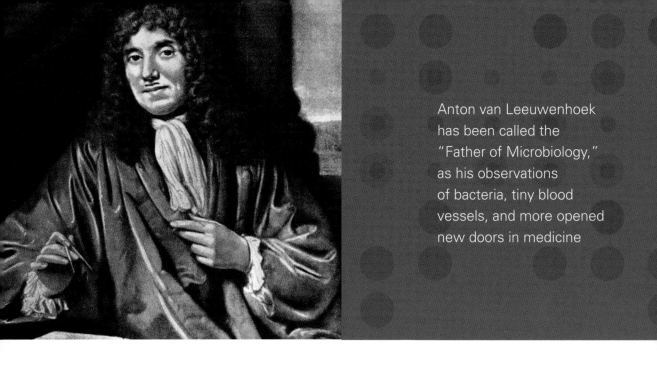

Anton van Leeuwenhoek has been called the "Father of Microbiology," as his observations of bacteria, tiny blood vessels, and more opened new doors in medicine

word "chemistry" comes from an old Greek name for Egypt, *Khemia*, or "land of black earth," so-called because of the fertile, crop-growing region found along the Nile River in Egypt.

During the Middle Ages, which lasted from approximately A.D. 476 to 1453, people remained unaware that living in dirty, crowded conditions directly contributed to health problems, and diseases such as leprosy, smallpox, and dysentery—an illness that causes severe diarrhea—were rampant. In the 1300s, a deadly disease called bubonic plague swept through Europe out of central Asia. The plague, which causes severely swollen lymph nodes, also known as buboes, usually originates with bacteria that live in the stomachs of fleas that feed on the blood of rats or other rodents. People develop the disease after being bitten by infected fleas, by handling animals with the disease, or by coming into contact with a person carrying it. The unsanitary living conditions in cities through-out much of Europe put many people in close proximity to fleas and rats, and the plague became an **epidemic**. From 1347 to 1351, bubonic plague, also called the Black Death, killed 25 million people, or about 1 out of every 4 people in the world. Doctors believed the best treatment for the plague was bloodletting—using leeches to drain blood from sick patients.

By the 1500s, scientists began to speculate that diseases were caused by tiny living creatures too small to see. An Italian physician

## THE MICROSCOPE SHEDS NEW LIGHT

*Historians often credit Hans and Zacharias Janssen, father and son lens makers from Holland, with inventing the microscope. In the 1590s, they noticed that objects appeared much closer when a person looked through two carefully shaped lenses in a straight line. This tool magnified objects 3 to 10 times, allowing researchers to view human tissues, cells, and the germs they had speculated about but could not previously see. Today, light microscopes, which use light to assist in the magnification, can enlarge views of tissue and blood samples up to 2,000 times. The most powerful of all are electron microscopes, which use beams of electrons—the negatively charged particles in atoms—instead of light to produce magnifications of a million times or more.*

named Girolamo Fracastoro studied various diseases, including smallpox, cholera, and the plague. In 1546, he suggested that tiny organisms, which he called "disease seeds," were responsible for illness. Fracastoro believed they could spread sickness through direct contact, through contaminated food or clothing, or through the air. Although his ideas were widely praised by scientists for a short time, his disease seeds soon were largely forgotten.

More than 100 years later, Dutch naturalist Anton van Leeuwenhoek made an important discovery. He was not a doctor or a trained scientist, but he enjoyed grinding glass lenses, assembling microscopes, and using them to look at small objects such as strands of hair and insect wings. Van Leeuwenhoek noticed tiny animals swimming in a single drop of water, and he called the creatures animalcules. He began to write letters about his findings to the Royal Society of London, a prominent group of scholars who discussed scientific matters. In one 1683 letter, van Leeuwenhoek detailed an experiment in which he took some plaque from his teeth and from four other people and compared the samples. "I then most always saw, with great wonder, that in the said matter there were many very little living animalcules, very prettily a-moving," he wrote in what was likely the first description of bacteria. Despite this huge medical discovery, scientists did not realize that animalcules had any connection to disease.

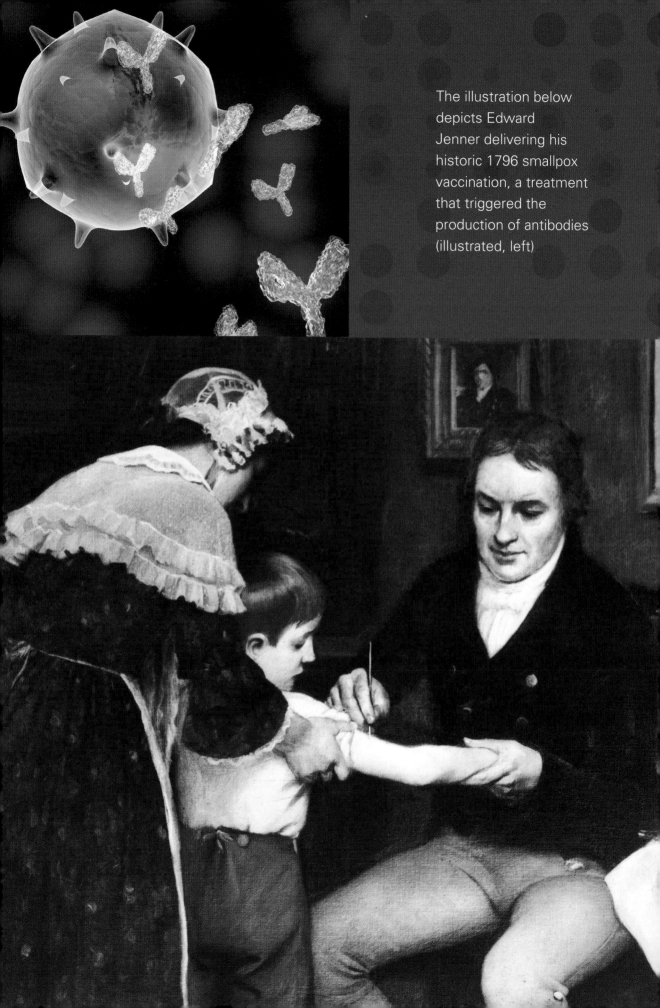

The illustration below depicts Edward Jenner delivering his historic 1796 smallpox vaccination, a treatment that triggered the production of antibodies (illustrated, left)

In 1796, an English doctor named Edward Jenner administered the first recorded **vaccination** to prevent a disease. Smallpox was a highly contagious and often lethal disease marked by chills, fever, hallucinations, and pus-filled sores. As a country doctor, Jenner had treated milkmaids for cowpox, a milder form of smallpox that was common in cows. The milkmaids contracted the disease from milking infected cows, but Jenner noticed that once they had recovered from cowpox, the women did not develop smallpox. Jenner drew pus from the sore of a patient with cowpox and injected it into the son of a local farmer. The boy developed cowpox, and after he recovered from the disease, Jenner intentionally infected the boy with smallpox. The boy did not develop smallpox. Although Jenner could not explain why his experiment worked, we now know that immunizations, which contain a dead or weakened form of a disease, cause a person's body to produce antibodies. These antibodies fight off the invading germs, and if the germs return, the antibodies recognize them and fight them again.

Finally, in the 1800s, several researchers began drawing connections between van Leeuwenhoek's animalcules and disease. Both French scientist Louis Pasteur and German physician Robert Koch studied germs of various diseases, including anthrax, and worked to develop vaccines. A Hungarian physician named Ignaz Semmelweis worked at a teaching hospital, where students would study **cadavers**—getting blood on their hands and coats—and then go directly to

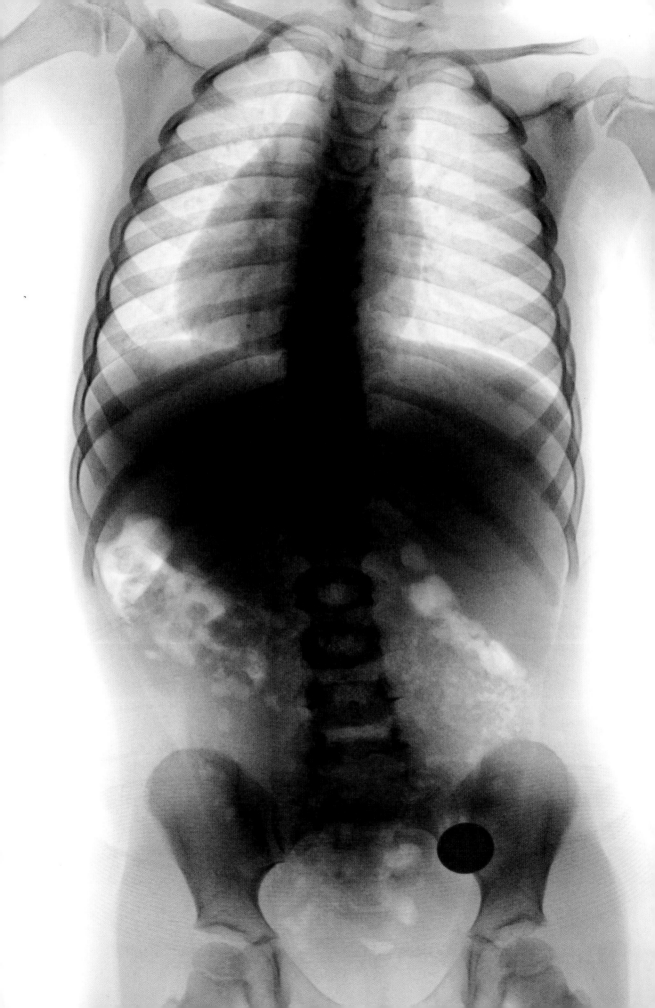

With X-rays, skeletal problems and foreign objects are shown clearly, as the images reveal the extent of bone breaks (right) or the location of a swallowed coin (opposite)

the maternity ward to deliver babies. In 1847, nearly one-third of the women who gave birth at the hospital developed an infection called childbed fever and died within a few days. Semmelweis came to believe childbed fever could be prevented if the doctors thoroughly washed their hands before visiting each patient. Indeed, once the routine was implemented, the rate of infections dropped dramatically.

As more germs were identified, researchers were able to develop drugs to fight them. Vaccinations helped prevent diseases, and antiseptics killed germs on doctors' hands and on medical instruments. Other drugs, such as penicillin, helped people recover from infections. Improved methods of infection prevention allowed physicians to perform surgeries more safely, with less risk of spreading germs to the patient's wound or internal organs. In 1895, German physicist Wilhelm Roentgen discovered a kind of electromagnetic radiation that he called X-rays. He found that these currents passed through soft tissues in the body but were blocked by bones and other hard surfaces. This discovery gave doctors a way to see inside

## CENTURIES OF SYRINGES

*Syringes—devices consisting of a piston inside a hollow cylinder—have been used in medicine for centuries. A book written by Greek inventor and mathematician Hero of Alexandria in the first century A.D. describes the use of syringes that can push out air or liquid. In ancient Greece, physicians used syringes mainly for drawing pus from boils and infected wounds; in fact, the Greek name for the syringe, pyulkos, means "pus puller." Physicians in the 1800s began to use syringes to inject medicine into a patient's tissues or muscle. Today, doctors and nurses use syringes every day to draw blood, give immunizations, or inject other medications.*

a patient's body to detect broken bones or any foreign objects, such as bullets or swallowed coins.

By the early 1950s, surgeons had operated on hearts, brains, and other major organs. The next advancement was organ transplantation—taking a healthy organ from one person and putting it inside a patient with a damaged or diseased organ. The first major organ transplants were done with kidneys, because although humans have two, they can live with just one functioning kidney. In the earliest cases, the kidney recipient began recovering after surgery, only to get sick again. British researcher Peter Medawar discovered that the problem was a physical reaction of the body called rejection. Patients receiving tissues from another person formed antibodies to fight off the new tissue, and the transplants failed. Joseph Murray, an American surgeon, confirmed this idea in 1954 when he performed a kidney transplant involving identical twin brothers. Because the donor's organ was not perceived by the body as foreign, the recipient's body accepted it.

Researchers then sought ways to help a patient's body accept foreign tissues. The drug cyclosporine was introduced in the 1970s as an effective immunosuppressant, a drug that prevents a patient's body from rejecting foreign tissue. Since then, kidney transplants have become safe and common procedures, paving the way for other organ transplant surgeries.

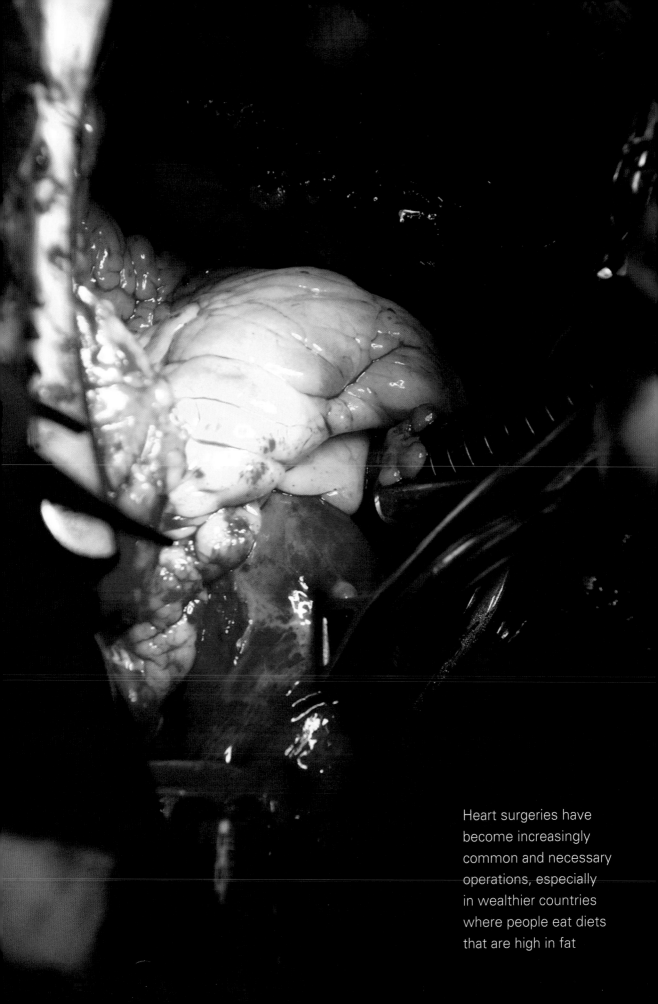

Heart surgeries have
become increasingly
common and necessary
operations, especially
in wealthier countries
where people eat diets
that are high in fat

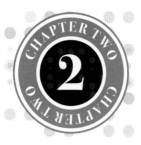
# TAKING THE FIGHT INWARD

In recent years, scientists have been studying cells and genes, the building blocks of our bodies, to find ways to cure diseases and extend lives. Researchers are also making gains in using robots to perform surgery and in using computers to help restore such functions as vision and physical movement in patients.

Researchers are particularly interested in stem cells. The human body is made up of billions of microscopic cells. We have blood cells, brain cells, and muscle cells, with each type performing a different job. If these cells die, they might not be replaced, and if too many cells die, that part of the body will be damaged. Stem cells are cells that can repair damage within our bodies by assuming the role of any kind of cell. For example, the stem cells in our skin replace skin cells damaged by a cut or sunburn. We can donate blood because the stem cells in our bone marrow will replace the lost blood cells. Researchers are today trying to figure out how to take these stem cells and put them in another person's body as a means of cell replacement. For years, doctors have performed bone marrow transplants, taking marrow cells from a healthy donor and putting them into a patient whose marrow is not working properly or has been damaged by invasive treatments such as **chemotherapy**. Scientists believe stem cells can help the body repair itself enough to recover from a variety of diseases, but the stem cells of adults generally do not adapt to other parts of the body.

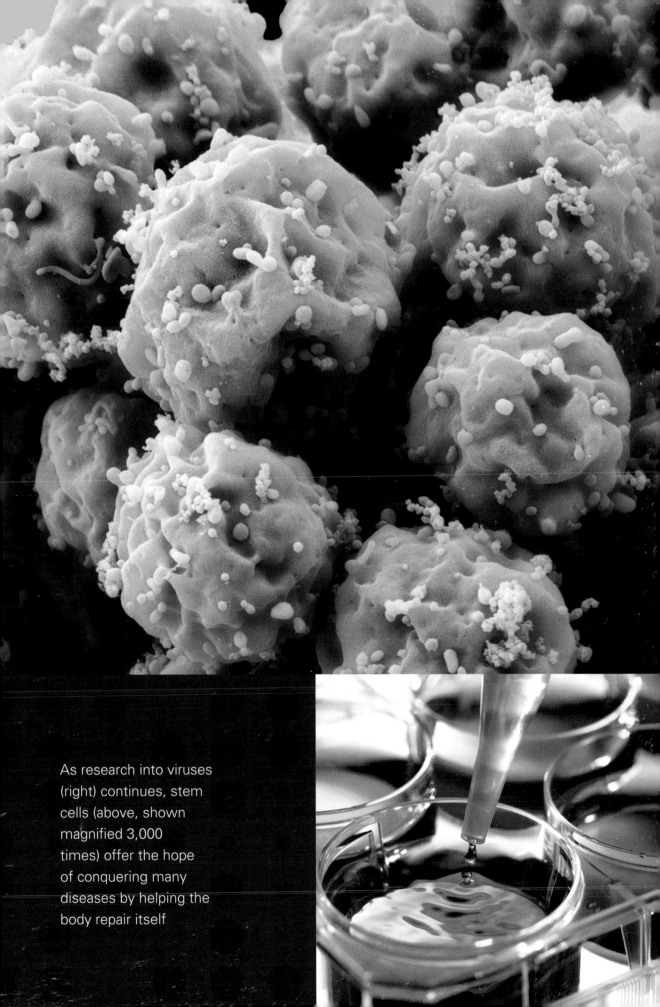

As research into viruses (right) continues, stem cells (above, shown magnified 3,000 times) offer the hope of conquering many diseases by helping the body repair itself

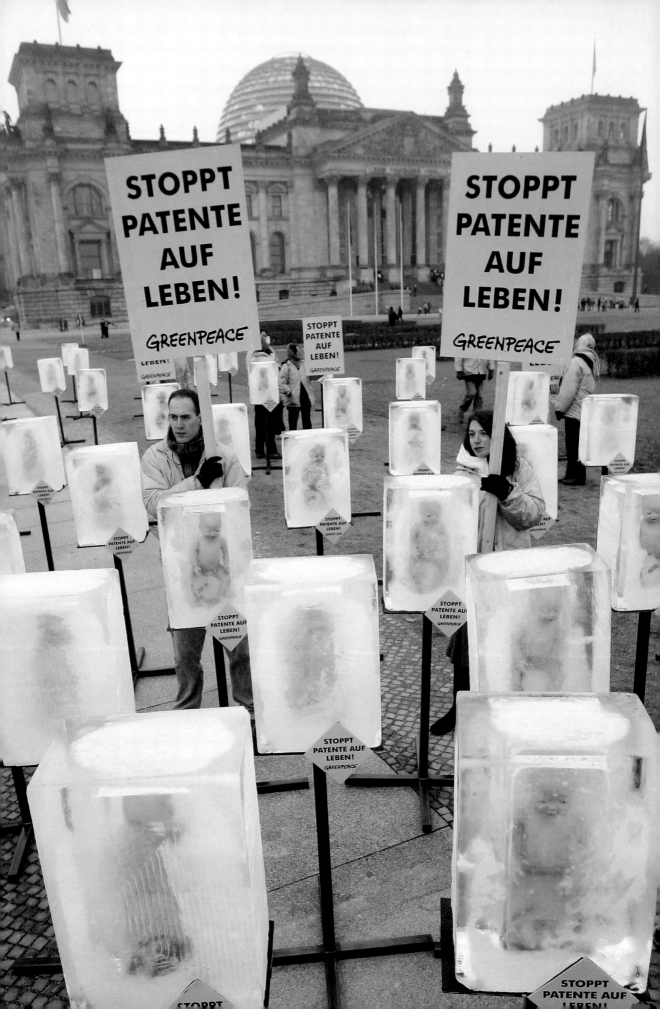

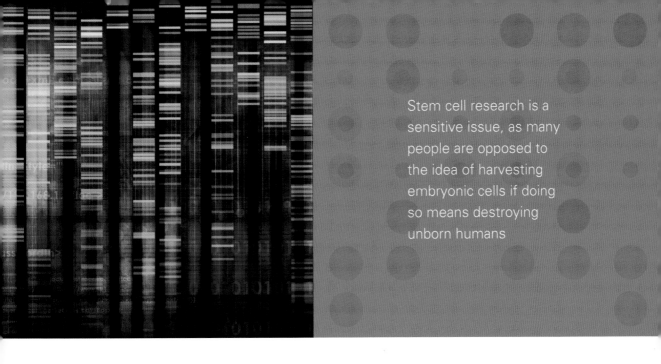

Stem cell research is a sensitive issue, as many people are opposed to the idea of harvesting embryonic cells if doing so means destroying unborn humans

Researchers have found a more adaptable stem cell in embryos, which are unborn humans in the very earliest stages of life. These embryonic stem cells have the potential to become any kind of cell, which has opened up possibilities for treating many diseases, including Alzheimer's disease, Parkinson's disease, and multiple sclerosis, which currently have no cure. Doing research with embryonic stem cells is highly controversial in the United States, however. Scientists obtain embryos from fertility clinics that would otherwise discard them because they no longer need them, and the harvesting of stem cells destroys the embryo. Many people oppose such stem cell research, believing it is morally wrong to deliberately destroy living embryos. Others fear that the use of embryonic stem cells might lead to people buying and selling embryos as "repair kits." Those in favor of the research point to the magnitude of possible benefits—conquering diseases and prolonging healthy lives.

Scientists are not only looking at transplanted cells as a means of fighting disease; they are also studying the "instructions" within cells. These instructions, called genes, form long strands of deoxy-ribonucleic acid, better known as DNA. Genes are **hereditary** and determine many aspects of our bodies, including eye color, hair color, height, and whether we are likely to develop certain diseases. In 2003, researchers for the Human Genome Project announced that they had fully mapped out the human genome—the roughly 20,500 genes in the human body. During the first decade of the 21st century, technology for genetic analysis improved, making the mapping process faster and cheaper.

Because of these advances, companies such as Navigenics, 23andMe, and deCODEme can today offer customers a look at their genetic map. Right now, this testing can reveal whether patients have an increased risk of developing diseases—for example, a specific type of cancer—that run in families. Genetic testing can indicate if chemotherapy is likely to help certain cancer patients. The test can even show whether a patient's cancer is likely to come back, or whether he or she has the gene for rare hereditary diseases. However, scientists say that, at present, the benefits of genetic mapping—which costs a patient about $10,000—are limited and won't lead to improved treatment for the average person. "Admittedly, right now your family history may be your best bet, and it doesn't cost anything," said Francis Collins, former director of the National Human Genome Research Institute.

Recent breakthroughs in medicine have also included ways to merge humans with machines to save and improve lives. In 2010, a

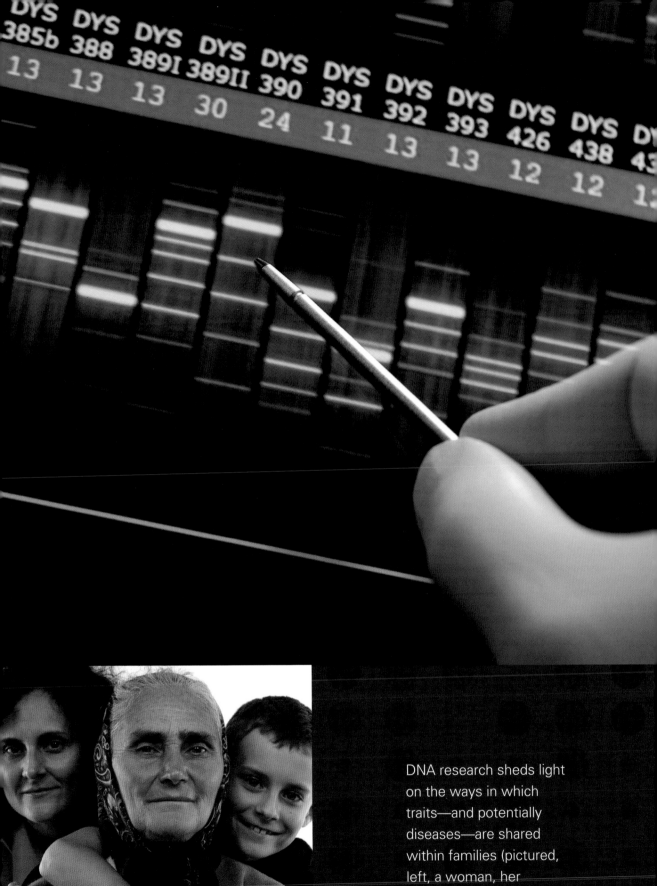

| DYS 385b | DYS 388 | DYS 389I | DYS 389II | DYS 390 | DYS 391 | DYS 392 | DYS 393 | DYS 426 | DYS 438 | DY 43 |
|---|---|---|---|---|---|---|---|---|---|---|
| 13 | 13 | 13 | 30 | 24 | 11 | 13 | 13 | 12 | 12 | 1 |

DNA research sheds light on the ways in which traits—and potentially diseases—are shared within families (pictured, left, a woman, her mother, and her son)

# LONGER LIVES AND BETTER HEALTH

*Medical advancements have been saving and improving lives for centuries, and people who become doctors aim to help individual patients and society as a whole. From advocating the use of clean water to developing immunizations and life-saving surgeries, researchers have helped people to live longer. Around A.D. 400, when the Roman Empire was ending, the average life expectancy was roughly 30 years. Although some people lived long lives, many died during infancy or childhood. In some **developed countries**, life expectancy has risen from 57 years in the early 1900s to more than 80 years today.*

43-year-old American named Charles Okeke received the first portable artificial heart machine, which runs on batteries and weighs about 13 pounds (5.9 kg). Before the operation, Okeke was connected to a 400-pound (181 kg) machine that kept his heart pumping, but improvements in technology allowed researchers to make a small device with enough power to support the heart. Okeke's ventricles—the two main chambers of the heart responsible for pumping blood to the entire body—and four of his heart valves were removed, and tubes connected the artificial heart in his chest to a power pack that he carried on his back.

A growing trend in modern surgery is using robots as surgeons. In the early 2000s, robots began helping doctors perform surgeries on the heart, brain, prostate, and other body parts. In robotic surgery, a robot is in the operating room with the patient, holding the necessary tools. A human surgeon sits in a different room, controlling the robot via remote controls and watching the procedure on a monitor. Canada's McGill University Health Centre took robotic surgery even farther in October 2010 when robots, controlled by doctors, both administered **anesthesia** and performed an operation in which a patient's prostate was removed. Experts say that robotic surgery offers many benefits over operations performed purely by human hands. The robots are programmed to make specific cuts, and their "hands" will never

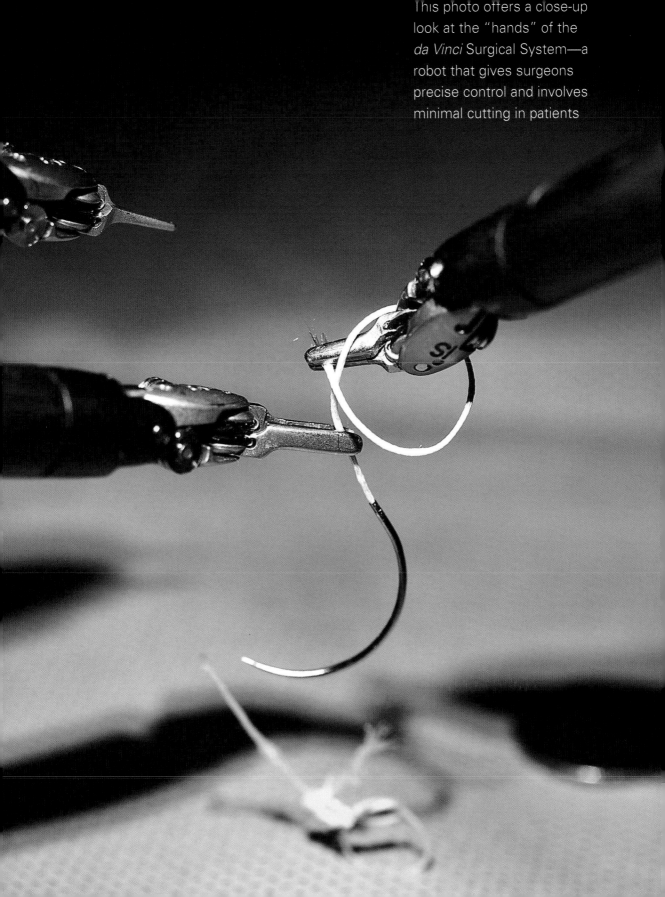
This photo offers a close-up look at the "hands" of the *da Vinci* Surgical System—a robot that gives surgeons precise control and involves minimal cutting in patients

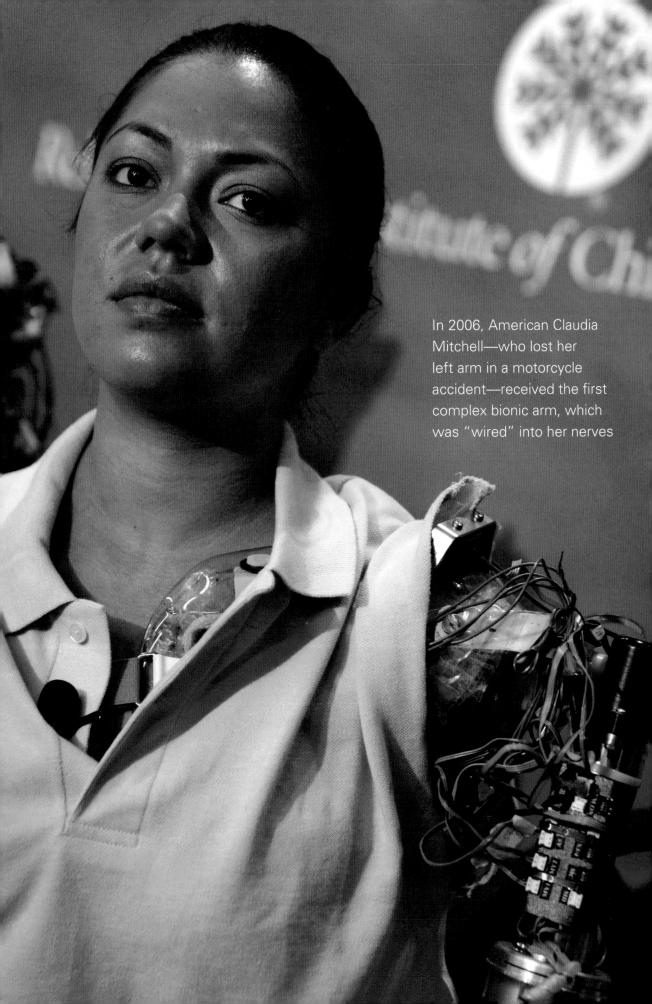

In 2006, American Claudia Mitchell—who lost her left arm in a motorcycle accident—received the first complex bionic arm, which was "wired" into her nerves shake or cut too deep. Surgical robots also can operate through smaller incisions, which improves patient safety and allows for faster recovery after the procedure.

The portable heart and the robotic surgeon are two ways in which machines have improved medicine. Another way is through bionics, or the use of mechanical and computerized systems to help patients regain lost movement, vision, and hearing. In the past, people who lost an arm or leg might be given a wooden, metal, or plastic **prosthesis** to take the place of the missing limb. But now, scientists are developing neural prostheses, which respond to commands from the patient's brain.

When people have a limb amputated, or removed, they might feel as if the arm or leg is still there. This sensation is called a phantom. In fact, the nerves leading to the lost limb are still alive but disconnected, like a telephone in a power outage. Todd Kuiken, a physician and biomedical engineer at the Rehabilitation Institute of Chicago, found a way to reroute these signals to different groups of muscles. Special sensors in a neural prosthesis are positioned over these muscles and are programmed to recognize the signals for particular movements. Then, the artificial arm sends the signals to a motor that drives mechanized parts to move the fingers, bend the elbow, or turn the wrist.

## A MEDICAL MISTAKE

*Improved medical treatment prevents people from getting sick and reduces the number of deaths from illnesses and injuries. But sometimes, new treatments can harm as well as help. In the 1950s, American scientist Jonas Salk developed a vaccine to protect people against polio, a disease that can cause paralysis and death. The vaccine was a success and was mass-produced for administration to schoolchildren. After the vaccination program began, some of the children got sick. Researchers discovered that a laboratory in California had not prepared the vaccine correctly. Although the vaccine protected thousands of children from polio, 200 developed the disease, and 11 died.*

Kuiken performed the procedure on Amanda Kitts, a woman who had lost the lower part of her left arm in a car accident, in 2006. "It was wonderful," Kitts said. "It made me feel more human because I could work it almost like a regular arm. I just had to think and it responded. My new arm made me feel like I could do anything again." While the human arm has more than 22 points of movement, a modern neural prosthesis can make only 7 movements. But in the next phase of improvements, researchers are hoping to create an arm capable of all 22 natural movements.

Researchers are also looking at computerized methods of restoring vision in people with **degenerative** eye diseases. After more than a decade of study and testing, scientists have come up with a way to use a tiny video camera and a computer to transmit video signals to 60 **electrodes** attached to the surface of the patient's retina, or the nerve layer that senses light at the back of the eye. This technology has not yet restored perfect vision, but it has allowed patients to see the outlines of objects again.

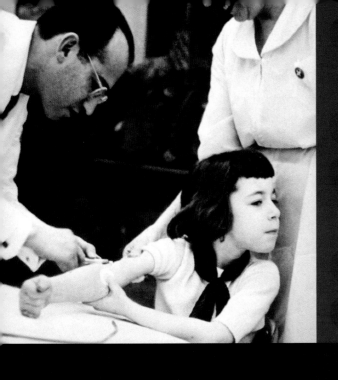

The polio vaccinations delivered by Jonas Salk (left) were a form of preventive medicine, while eye surgeries (below) represent corrective medicine

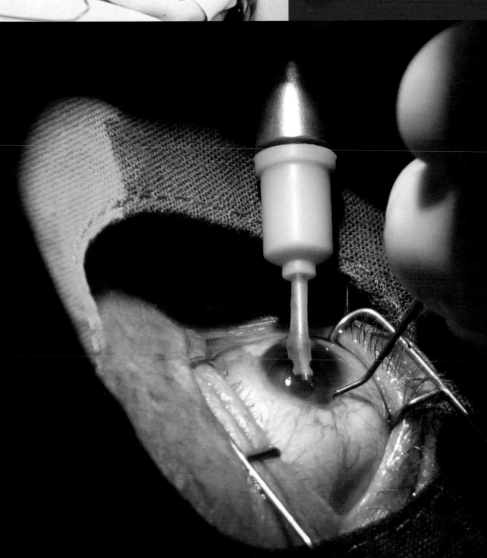

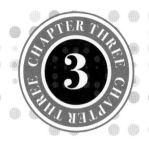

# CELLS AND SMALL SURGEONS

When you picture how medical procedures and treatments of the future will look, think small. By the middle of the 21st century, many treatments might work from the inside of the body in the form of new drugs and tiny robots that perform internal surgery. Such developments may one day make surgeries that require doctors to cut open the patient obsolete. For the most part, coming medical technologies will be aimed at keeping patients well rather than seeking out and reacting to diseases and disorders—prevention rather than cure.

Genetic testing will become more common as the price drops. Eventually, researchers predict, it will cost just $100 to map a person's genome in hours or minutes, compared with the $3 billion it cost for the first one to be completed from 1990 to 2003. "One could imagine that acquiring a complete genome sequence of an individual might become the standard of care one day," said Eric Green, director of the National Human Genome Research Institute.

As more people have their genes mapped, researchers will develop treatments tailored to the individual patient by looking at his or her genes. This genetic testing would reveal which health problems you are likely to encounter. It would also show which drugs would best work for you and would possibly allow the pharmacist to design a pill just for you—a pill that would prevent health problems, such as heart disease, diabetes, or certain types of cancer, from beginning. After receiving your genetic roadmap, you might visit with a doctor to discuss how your environment could affect

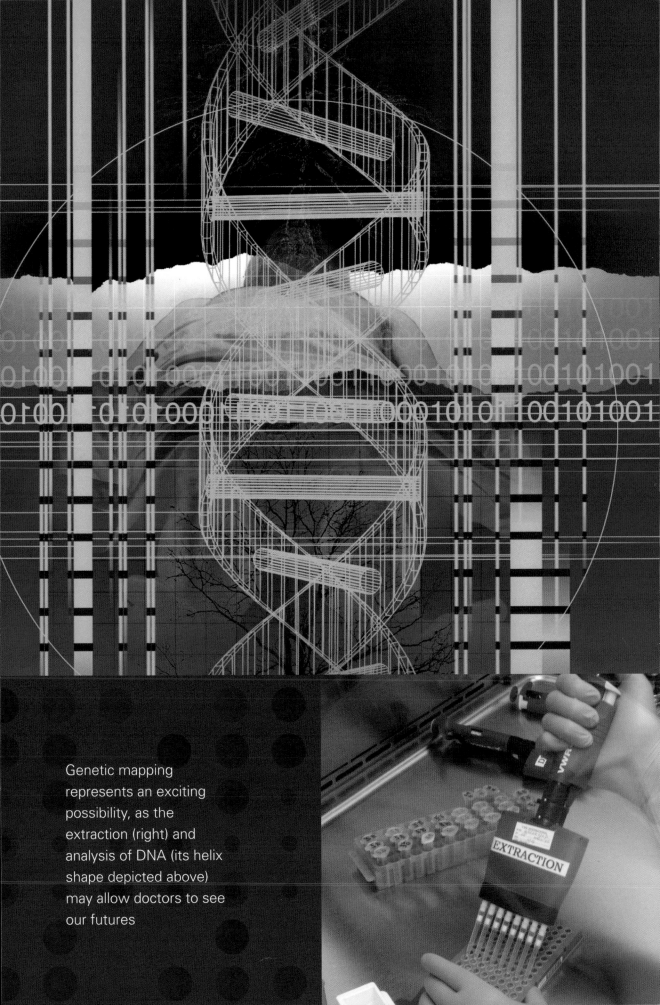

Genetic mapping represents an exciting possibility, as the extraction (right) and analysis of DNA (its helix shape depicted above) may allow doctors to see our futures

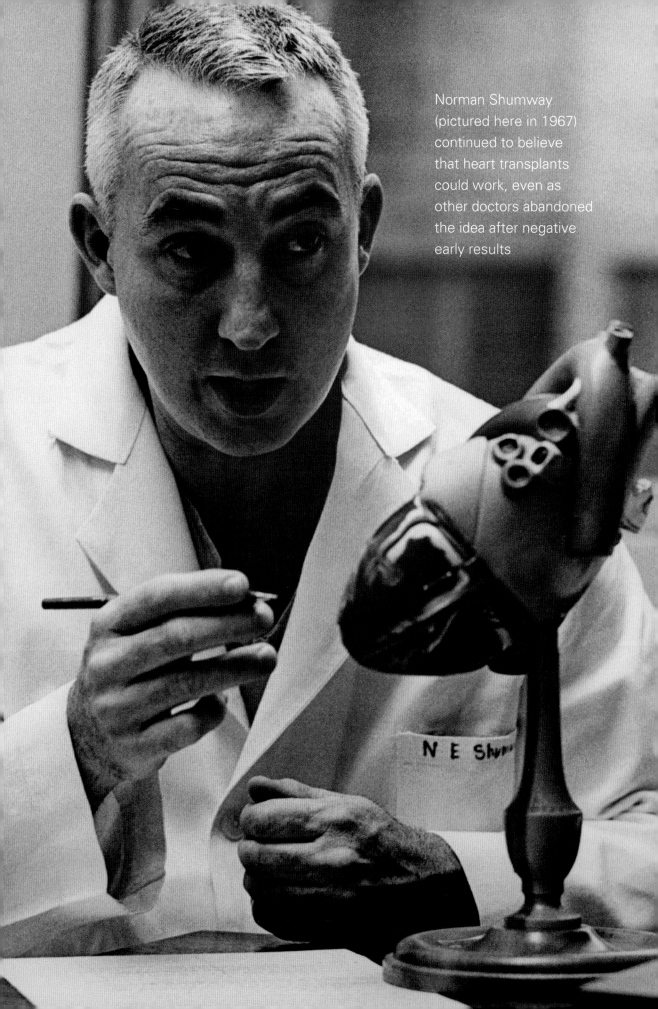

Norman Shumway (pictured here in 1967) continued to believe that heart transplants could work, even as other doctors abandoned the idea after negative early results

## THE TRANSPLANT AGE BEGINS

*On January 6, 1968, doctor Norman Shumway performed the first human-to-human heart transplant surgery in the U.S. During the next few years, many surgeons performed heart transplants, but the procedures were usually unsuccessful, with patients dying from complications after only a few days or weeks. Shumway began using a new drug called cyclosporine, which helped to keep patients from rejecting their new hearts. He also developed a procedure called a heart biopsy—removing a sample of tissue to check for disease—to treat a patient in the beginning stages of rejection before dangerous complications could arise. Today, most heart recipients live at least five years with their new organs.*

your genes, turning them on or off to cause diseases. Having this information would guide your lifestyle choices, such as the foods you eat or avoid. Or, for example, if your genes show that you are susceptible to developing skin cancer, you would know to take extra precautions in protecting your skin from the sun's radiation.

Genetics could also factor largely into future organ transplants. Scientists could take cells from newborns and store them for future use. If that child needed a new kidney or heart later in life, researchers could grow a new organ from the cells collected at birth. The patient's body would accept the organ because it came from the patient's own cells, avoiding the problem of rejection that many transplant patients experience today.

For people who had already developed clogged arteries or other forms of heart disease, medicine might be available to help grow new arteries and healthy heart muscle, eliminating the need for surgery. The doctor would inject drugs, either based on or made from stem cells, into the bloodstream. These drugs would travel to the heart and turn off the gene that prevents new cell growth. In heart attack patients, the cells would form new heart muscle to replace the cells that died from lack of oxygen. Within a few weeks, the patient's heart could be back to normal. In the same way, this type of drug could stimulate the growth of nerve cells to cure multiple sclerosis, brain cells to help **stroke** victims, or cells in the retina to reverse **macular degeneration**.

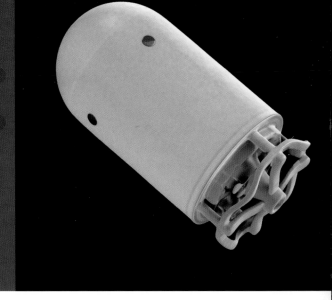

Cloning is a futuristic
development that has
already happened (Dolly
the sheep pictured,
opposite), and medical
nanobots (illustrated,
right) may be coming

In the future, patients who need surgery could undergo a procedure without any incisions being made on the outside of their bodies. First, the doctor would scan the patient's body to find the area in need of medical treatment. This scanning could be done with a small, handheld MRI (magnetic resonance imaging) device, about the size of a camera, instead of current MRI machines, which take up a small room. If the patient needed surgery, a robot called ARES (Assembling Reconfigurable Endoluminal Surgical system) might do the job from inside the patient's body. How would it get there? The patient would swallow up to 15 pill-sized pieces that would move through the body until they reached the surgery site and then assemble themselves into a working robot. Each piece would have a specific role to play in the surgery, such as communicating with a computer outside the body, taking diagnostic measurements, making incisions, and taking samples to be examined after the surgery. After an ARES operation, the patient would recover more quickly and with less pain than after traditional surgery because there would be fewer cuts to heal. The robot would either **disintegrate** in the body or follow the digestive system and leave the body naturally.

Even smaller robots and treatments will come from the field of nanotechnology. Nanotechnology involves structures that are so tiny they can interact with individual cells inside the body. A nanometer is one-billionth of a meter, a size so small it cannot be

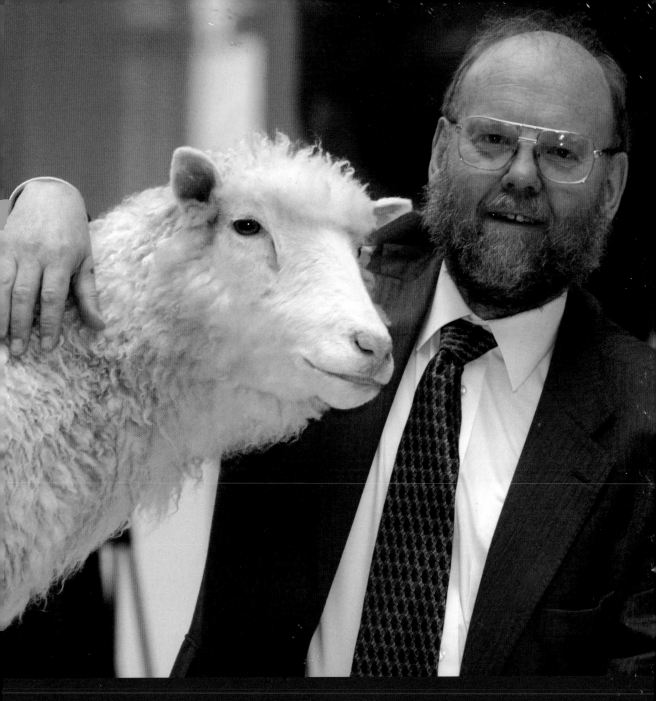

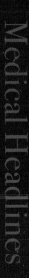

## THE CONTROVERSY OF CLONING

**Cloning** is a major source of controversy in medical research today. In the 1990s, researchers in Scotland cloned a sheep and created Dolly, a sheep that was identical to the original animal. The success of this experiment led to serious debates. Scientists believe that this technology may allow them to someday produce organs for transplant surgeries and healthy cells to replace the damaged ones in people with Alzheimer's or Parkinson's disease. But there are problems, too. Scientists have found that cloned animals, such as mice and cows, are prone to higher-than-normal rates of infection, disease, and tumors. Some people also feel it is unethical for scientists to have such control over human life.

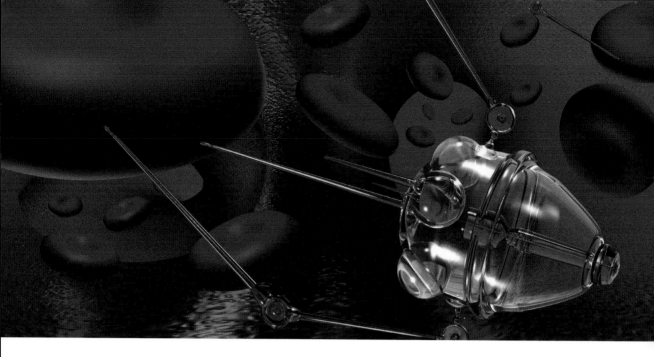

seen with any microscope yet developed. Equipped with cameras and sensors, tiny robots called nanobots will one day allow doctors to see how cells act inside the body and whether abnormal or diseased cells are present. Researchers predict many benefits of nanomedicine, and some even believe that medical pain and many common diseases, such as heart disease and infections, will no longer exist by the middle of the 21st century.

Today, when cancer patients undergo chemotherapy to kill their cancerous cells, the drugs kill some of their healthy cells, too. Nanotechnology could help deliver the necessary drugs without hurting healthy cells. To fight cancer, nanobots may one day search for cancerous cells. When they find one, they would analyze it and destroy it with a poison released to kill just that cell. If no cancer cells are detected, the nanobots would travel through the body as tiny guardians. People would no longer worry about their cancer returning, since, as soon as cancer cells began to form, the nanobots would detect and destroy them. Similarly, the nanobots might roam a patient's bloodstream, acting as an artificial **immune system** to identify infections and viruses. They would act more quickly than the body's regular white blood cells, and they could be programmed to fight new diseases. Nanobots could potentially also perform the most delicate surgeries, such as operating on a fetus, or unborn child, still in the womb.

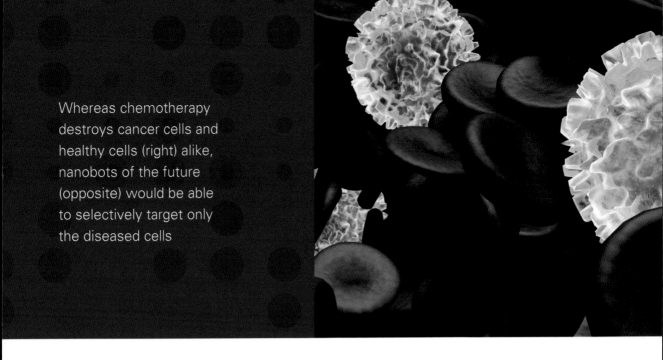

Whereas chemotherapy destroys cancer cells and healthy cells (right) alike, nanobots of the future (opposite) would be able to selectively target only the diseased cells

Another use for nanomedicine may be in protecting our bodies against accident or injury. Having nanobots permanently placed in a person's skin could make the skin stronger, more resistant to tearing, and faster healing. Mixing nanomaterials with the body's cells could speed the regrowth of broken bones. Placed in a person's **glands**, nanobots might have the capability to jumpstart **hormone** production. Various hormone levels in our bodies decline as we age, and if nanobots could increase our hormone levels, they could reverse the effects of aging, and we might look and feel younger.

Nanotechnology is also helping bionics move forward. Some researchers predict that in as little as two decades, artificial limbs will be covered with artificial skin able to sense temperature and touch. Ultra-thin carbon nanotubes, only 1/10,000th as thick as a human hair, would cover the skin in the same way that human hair grows from skin and function to conduct heat and electricity to a person's nerves. This technology might also help replace damaged skin in burn victims.

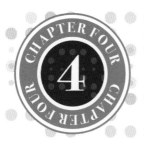

# SCIENCE FICTION TO MEDICAL FACT

Avoiding disease with a gene repair or having tiny machines swimming through our bodies in search of cancerous cells seem like story lines from a science-fiction movie. However, scientists believe that with years of research and steady advancements in technology, they can overcome potential problems or fears about these new types of treatment, making them standard practices in the medical community.

Many genetic diseases are caused by problems in more than one gene. Sometimes, environmental factors can trigger the genes to cause diseases. To better understand how this happens, researchers in several countries, including Sweden and the United Kingdom (UK), have recruited thousands of volunteers for their **biobanks**. In the UK, more than 450,000 people have agreed to donate their DNA and have their medical records tracked for the rest of their lives. The principal investigator for the project, Rory Collins, professor of medicine and **epidemiology** at Oxford University, said that to find out how genes work together and work with the environment, "you need to do studies that are very, very big. It's only just now that the technology allows those experiments to be done."

Armed with enough blood samples to fill two tanker trucks and the promise of being able to track changes as volunteers return for future checkups, researchers hope to unlock the secrets behind widespread medical problems such as arthritis, heart disease, and diabetes. They hope the results will reveal trends in how a person's environment—which includes what people eat, where they work, the

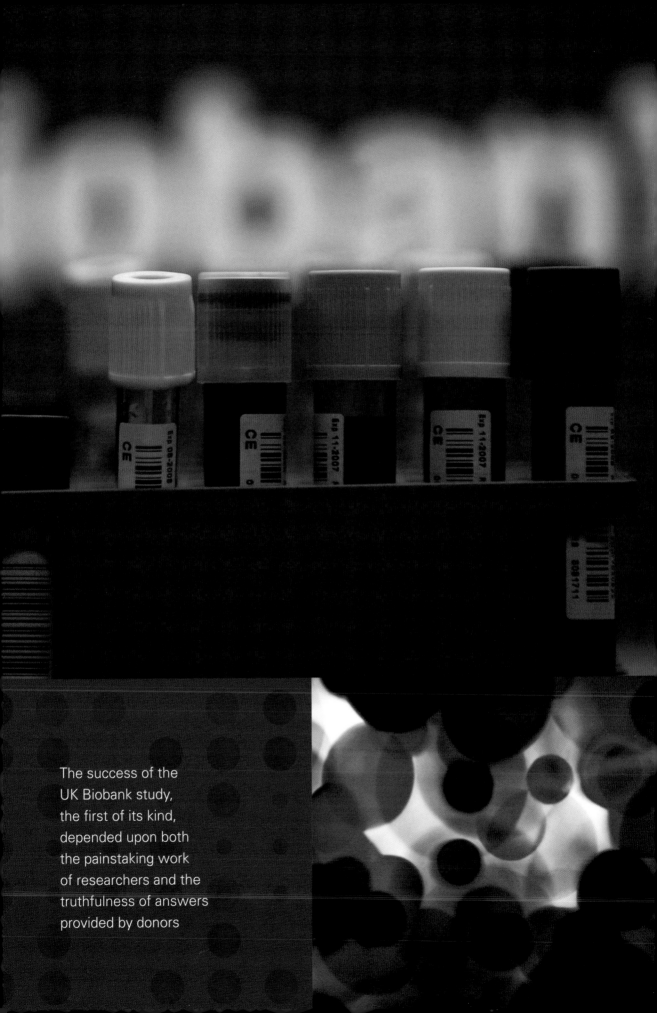

The success of the
UK Biobank study,
the first of its kind,
depended upon both
the painstaking work
of researchers and the
truthfulness of answers
provided by donors

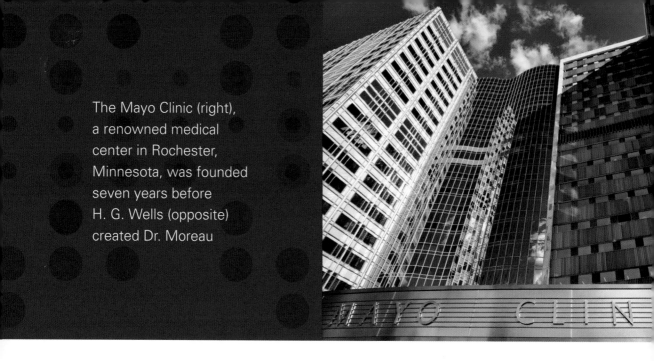

The Mayo Clinic (right), a renowned medical center in Rochester, Minnesota, was founded seven years before H. G. Wells (opposite) created Dr. Moreau

pollution or chemicals to which they are exposed, and other factors—may impact the development of diseases. In the U.S., the Mayo Clinic began collecting blood and tissue samples in 2009 as part of a 3-year project to enroll 20,000 of its patients for ongoing study.

The problem with collecting enormous quantities of data is that the human brain, and even today's fastest computers, cannot sort and fully analyze all of it. Machines that sequence the human genome produce trillions of bits of data. Before gene mapping becomes a common practice in health care, it will need to be quick and easy to do, and the results must have clear meaning for doctors and patients. In the future, researchers hope that computer programs will be able to glean all the information from a genome and neatly summarize it. Much progress has already been made since the first genome was sequenced. Researchers spent 13 years creating that map. With new companies competing to perfect gene mapping, and with improvements in computer capabilities, a genome sequence in 2011 could be done in just over a week.

To make nanomachines a reality, scientists will need to figure out how to take the obvious but challenging first step—building them. Today, researchers are attempting to develop the various parts of nanodevices. The National Institutes of Health has created the Nanomedicine Roadmap Initiative, and eight development centers are studying how cells and molecules operate to understand how nanodevices will interact with them. Nanobots will need much

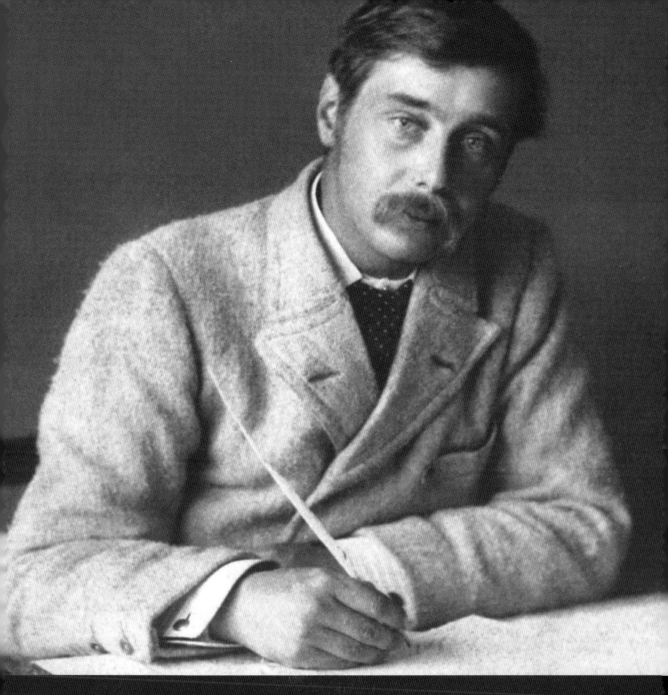

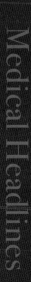
## WELLS FORESHADOWS GENETIC EXPERIMENTS

*In 1896, English science-fiction author H. G. Wells wrote* The Island of Dr. Moreau. *In the novel, the mysterious Dr. Moreau lives on a secluded island, where he performs vivisections, or operations on live animals, to create half-human, half-animal creatures. Although such studies have never been legitimately done in real life, scientists have used animals in medical research and testing for many years. Tropical fish have been genetically altered to glow in the dark. Cattle, sheep, goats, and pigs have been used in cloning experiments. Researchers have investigated ways to change the genes of these animals so that they will produce human* **proteins** *that might one day be used for medicine.*

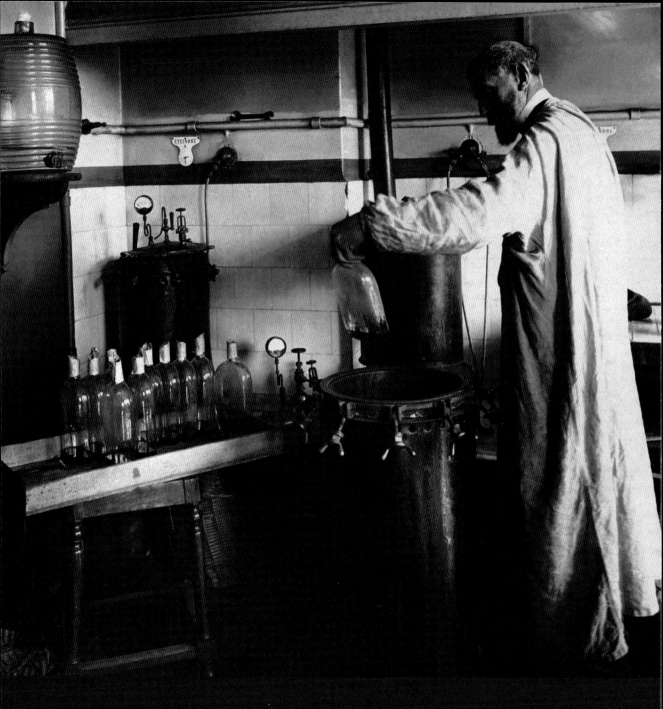

## PASTEUR'S GERM-KILLING PROCESS

*During the 19th century, while scientists were beginning to believe that germs caused disease, a French chemist and microbiologist named Louis Pasteur was devising a way to kill germs. He believed that if doctors boiled their medical instruments and steamed the bandages, the heat would destroy the germs on the objects and reduce infections among patients. He applied his ideas to perishable foods and also discovered that sealing containers shut bacteria out. His process of heating (mostly liquid) foods to kill bacteria became known as pasteurization, and it is still used to extend the shelf life of milk, orange juice, and other foods.*

smaller and faster computers than are currently available. Instead of building computers out of silicon chips as they do now, researchers might use nanochips, built atom by atom. It is a daunting process, but each year brings new advances. Just a few decades ago, a single computer filled an entire room; today, such a machine would be dwarfed in power by a computer smaller than a notebook. It is therefore not a stretch to think that nanocomputers will become a reality in the not-so-distant future.

Because nanobots will be so incredibly small, it could take millions of them to perform the tasks for which they are designed. Rather than building each one, scientists might design nanobots so that they can **replicate** themselves. How big should they be, and how fast should they move? Nanobots will need a source of energy to perform their jobs, and researchers have yet to figure out how to power such microscopic machines.

Despite the potential advantages of nanomedicine and other medical advances, patients might not embrace these new kinds of treatment. Scientists will need to consider and overcome the dangers and ethical dilemmas posed by these areas of research. For example, if nanobots are designed to multiply inside the body, what if they don't stop? What happens if they quit working? Also, some people might worry that if these technologies can be used to help, they could also be used to cause damage and might be put to sinister uses. Could nanobots be designed to dismantle blood cells, bones, or organs, one molecule at a time—essentially becoming terrifying weapons?

Like nanomedicine, genetic manipulation is a controversial area of research marked by many questions. Many researchers and cor- porations today are attempting to improve plants, animals, and food with genetic engineering. They have made certain crops resistant to disease, and they have modified the genes of some cows so that

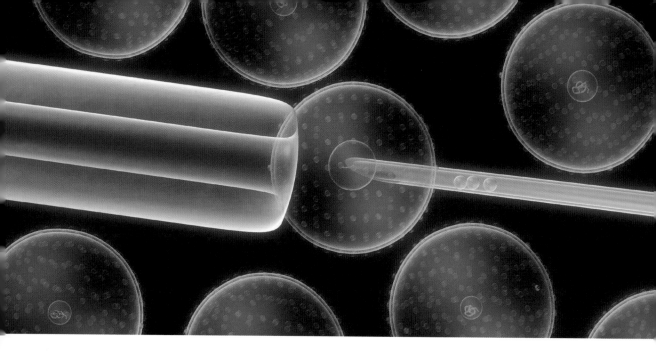

the animals produce more milk, or milk with different nutrients in it. But experiments in gene research can also lead to mistakes, including potentially fatal ones. In 2001, a group of scientists created a genetically modified virus to keep mice from having babies. Instead, the virus killed the mice. Scientists someday could intentionally create genetically modified viruses specifically designed to harm people. If countries develop such bioweapons, warfare will become even more dangerous.

Some experts are against modifying human genes and using stem cells for ethical reasons. Once scientists are able to "fix" genes to help people avoid getting sick, they will probably be able to identify specific genes that parents want for their babies. Of course, no one wants their children to develop diseases, but how much control is too much? Should parents be able to create "designer babies," choosing their child's genes to maximize their appearance, intelligence, or athletic ability? Also, when a patient has his or her genome mapped in the future, it will likely reveal the natural causes that may lead to the person's death. Employers who have access to such information about potential employees might not hire certain people. Insurance companies might refuse to offer coverage to people depending on their predicted cause of death. Countries will need to establish regulations for dealing with these complicated issues.

Regardless of whether researchers use adult or embryonic stem cells, they will need to further their studies before this

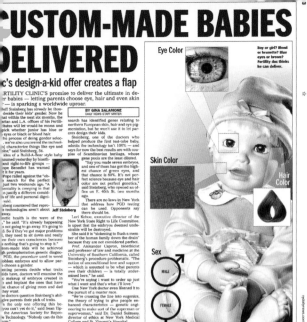

# CUSTOM-MADE BABIES DELIVERED

## c's design-a-kid offer creates a flap

**Eye Color**

**Skin Color**

**Hair Color**

**Sex** — MALE / FEMALE

While the ability to manipulate cells (illustrated, opposite) could be a life-saving development, it could also cause disputes about how much control people should have over such matters

treatment can be considered a safe option. Studies of stem cells injected into mice and other test animals have shown that the stem cells that do not migrate to the desired location in the body can build up in other areas and form cancerous tumors. Researchers will also need to find better ways of preventing the body from attacking unrecognized cells and tissues taken from other people.

Before doctors can treat the general public with new drugs or medical devices, the treatments must be proved safe and effective. In the U.S., the Food and Drug Administration (FDA) oversees medical technologies and approves the ones that meet specific standards. New treatments must go through many rounds of testing, which could take months or years to complete. Still, with research already underway in many areas, medicine could be much different in 20 years from what it is today. Doctors will need to be prepared to use the latest advances in medicine, which means that medical universities will need to alter their methods of instructing new generations of doctors.

The field of medicine has advanced rapidly in the past 500 years. Today, in the early years of the 21st century, scientists are looking at medicine with a new purpose. No longer content merely to understand and treat diseases, many now aspire to be able to prevent disease with genetic mapping and nanorobotic mainte- nance. Although numerous hurdles remain to realizing such fan- tastic medical know-how, the world of medicine will undoubtedly change, and perhaps sooner than we think.

43

# GLOSSARY

**anesthesia** — a drug that makes a patient lose sensation or consciousness before a surgery begins

**archaeologists** — scientists who study material remains such as artifacts, monuments, and bones to learn about past human life and activities

**biobanks** — collections of stored biological materials, such as human tissue or blood samples, and clinical information about the donors of the materials

**cadavers** — dead bodies intended for dissection as part of scientific study

**chemotherapy** — the treatment of a disease (usually cancer) using chemicals or drugs that selectively destroy diseased cells or whatever is causing the disease

**cloning** — the process of creating one or more genetic duplicates of a single organism by artificial or controlled means

**degenerative** — describing a condition that causes the body or part of the body to become weaker or less able to function as time passes

**developed countries** — the wealthiest countries of the world, which are generally characterized by good health care, nutrition, education, and industry

**disintegrate** — to break into many small parts or pieces

**electrodes** — conductors through which an electric current enters or leaves a substance; they can be used to detect electrical activity, such as brain waves, in the body

**epidemic** — an occurrence in which a disease spreads very quickly and affects a large number of people

**epidemiology** — the study of patterns of health and illness and factors associated with health in a given population

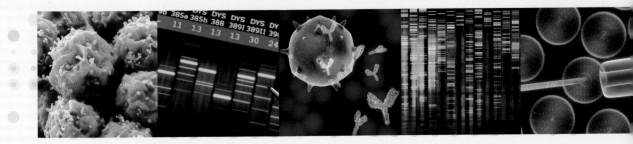

**genes** — hereditary units that determine the particular characteristics of an organism

**glands** — organs in the body that draw certain substances from blood and alter them into new substances that help the body function

**hereditary** — describing traits that are passed from parents to children before birth

**hormone** — a natural substance that is produced in the body and that influences the way the body grows or develops

**immune system** — the collection of biological structures (such as white blood cells) and processes that a body uses to fight disease

**incision** — a cut made into a body during surgery

**laxatives** — food or drugs that stimulate bowel movements

**macular degeneration** — a gradual loss of the central part of a person's field of vision, usually affecting both eyes and occurring especially in the elderly

**parasitic** — describing an organism that grows and feeds on or in a different organism while contributing nothing to its host

**prosthesis** — an artificial device that replaces or assists a missing or impaired part of the body

**proteins** — substances responsible for the growth and repair of tissues in human and animal bodies

**replicate** — to duplicate, or produce an identical or near-identical copy

**stroke** — a serious medical condition caused by the sudden stoppage of blood flow to the brain; it can result in long-term brain damage or physical problems

**vaccination** — the administration of a specially prepared dose of tiny organisms such as viruses as a means of making the body increase its ability to fight a particular disease

# SELECTED BIBLIOGRAPHY

Claybourne, Anna. *The Usborne Introduction to Genes & DNA*. London: Usborne Publishing, 2006.

Fischman, Josh. "A Better Life with Bionics." *National Geographic*, January 2010.

Fox, Maggie, Julie Steenhuysen, and Ben Hirschler. "Special Report: Fast Machines, Genes and the Future of Medicine." *Reuters.com*, March 30, 2010. http://www.reuters.com/assets/ print?aid=USTRE62T0KC20100330.

Hanson, William. *The Edge of Medicine: The Technology That Will Change Our Lives*. New York: Palgrave Macmillan, 2008.

Herbst, Judith. *Germ Theory*. Minneapolis: Twenty-First Century Books, 2008.

Schimpff, Stephen. *The Future of Medicine: Megatrends in Health Care That Will Improve Your Quality of Life*. Nashville: Thomas Nelson, 2007.

Woods, Michael, and Mary B. Woods. *Ancient Medicine: From Sorcery to Surgery*. Minneapolis: Runestone Press, 2000.

# WEB SITES

**HowStuffWorks: How Designer Children Work**
*http://science.howstuffworks.com/environmental/life/genetic/ designer-children.htm*
This site provides a detailed but accessible explanation of the human genome and discusses how genetic mapping may make it possible for parents to "design" children.

**UK Biobank**
*http://www.ukbiobank.ac.uk/*
Learn more about the UK Biobank study at this site. Among other topics, it explains how a giant freezer facility was built to store the study's 10 million blood samples.

# INDEX

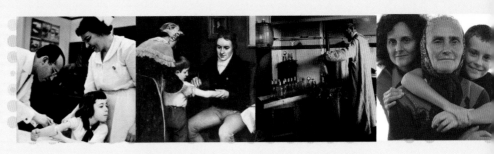

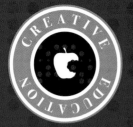

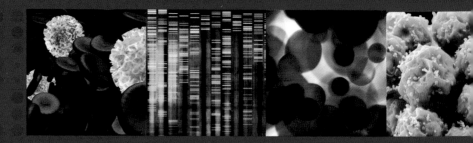

Published by Creative Education
P.O. Box 227, Mankato, Minnesota 56002
Creative Education is an imprint of The Creative Company
www.thecreativecompany.us

Design and production by The Design Lab
Art direction by Rita Marshall
Printed in the United States of America

Photographs by Alamy (AF Archive, Everett Collection Inc., INTERFOTO, Mic Smith
Photography LCC, Jeremy Sutton-Hibbert), Bigstock (biopic, danilo2, Eraxion, Flogel,
kentoh, krishnacreations), Corbis (Bettmann/Corbis, Steve Gschmeissner/Science
Photo Library, Hulton-Deutsch Collection/Corbis, Jason Reed/Reuters), Dreamstime
(Alexstar, Billyfoto, Cornelius20, Diego Vito Cervo, Vasily Kaleda, Stanislav Perov,
Pictureguy66, Pseudolongino, Nurbek Sagynbaev, Skyhawk911, Serghei Starus, Tallik,
Xalanx), Getty Images (Christopher Furlong, Sean Gallup, NY Daily News Archive,
Popperfoto), iStockphoto (dra_schwartz, Gunnar Assmy, Pgiam)

Library of Congress Cataloging-in-Publication Data

Dittmer, Lori.
The future of medicine / by Lori Dittmer.
p. cm. — (What's next?)
Summary: A look at potential future developments in medicine, including the use of
nanotechnology, as well as genetic mapping and other technologies that are currently
considered state-of-the-art.
Includes bibliographical references and index.
ISBN 978-1-60818-222-0
1. Medicine—Juvenile literature. 2. Medicine—Forecasting—Juvenile literature.
3. Medical innovations—Juvenile literature. I. Title.

R130.5.D58 2013
610.28—dc23      2011040507

First edition

9 8 7 6 5 4 3 2 1

*Cover: A digital illustration of the influenza virus*
*Page 1: A hospital patient being X-rayed in 1933*
*Page 2: A digital illustration of DNA data*

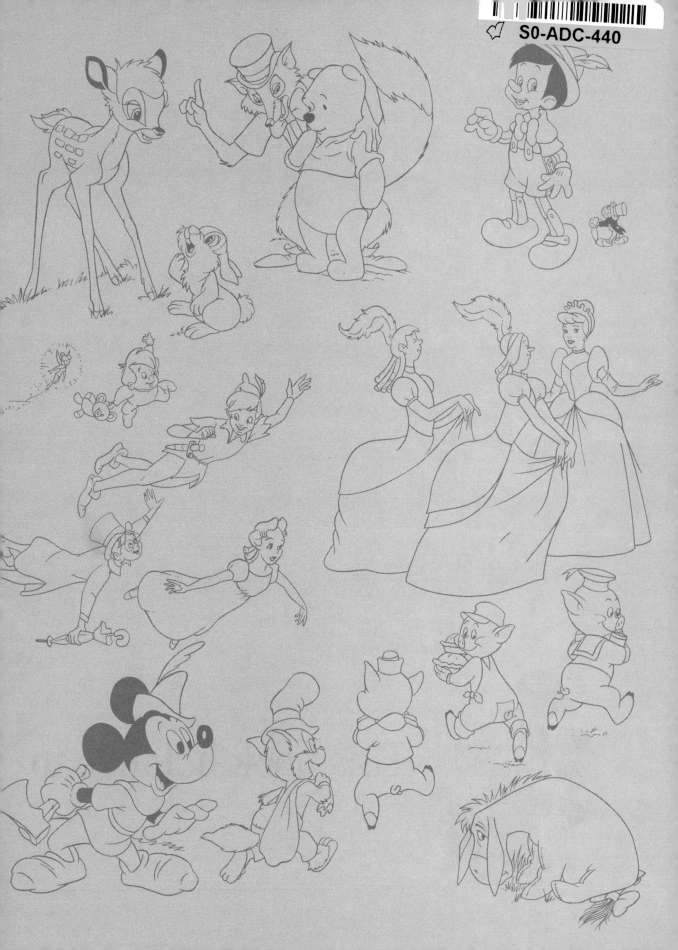

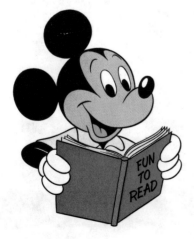

# This book belongs to

_____

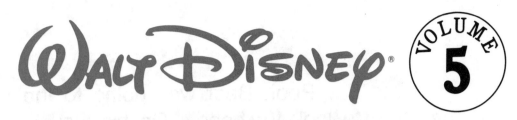

# POOH'S
# NEW CLOTHES

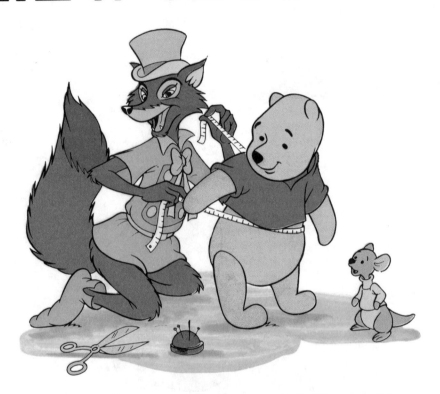

WALT DISNEY **FUN-TO-READ** LIBRARY

ISBN 1-885222-17-3
Advance Publishers Inc., P.O. Box 2607, Winter Park, FL. 32790
Printed in the United States of America
098765432

One day Pooh Bear was going to the bee tree to look for honey. On his way he saw a surprising thing. All of his friends were together in one place.

"Dear, dear!" said Pooh. "I wonder what is going on."

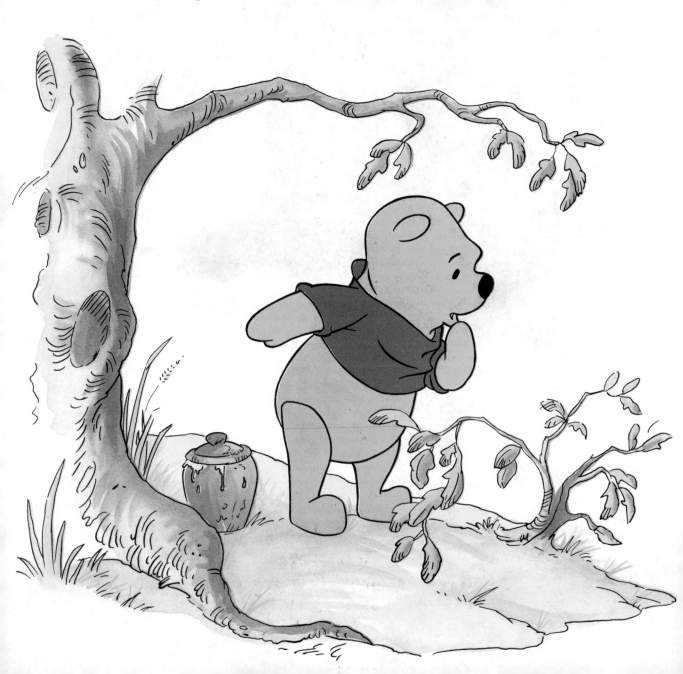

Then through the crowd he saw a fox.
"Who could he be?" Pooh wondered.
"Well, I'll just take a look and see!"

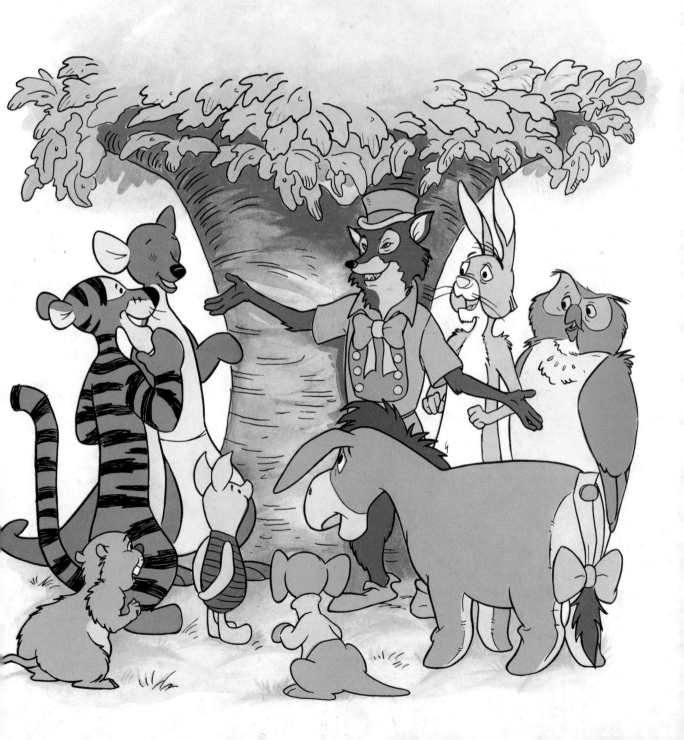

In the center of the crowd stood the handsome fox. The fox held up one beautiful outfit after another.

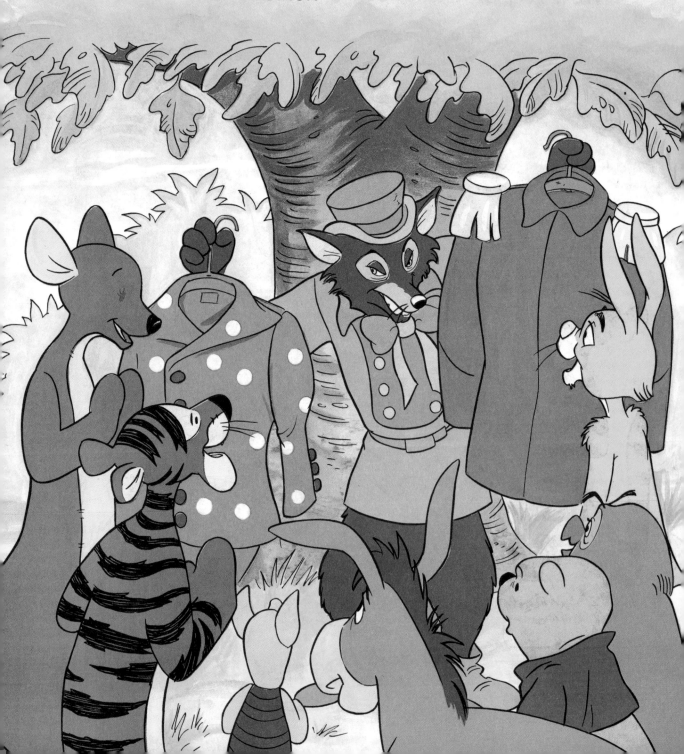

"Only someone who is very important would ever wear clothes like these. Take it from me, Sly Fox," said he.

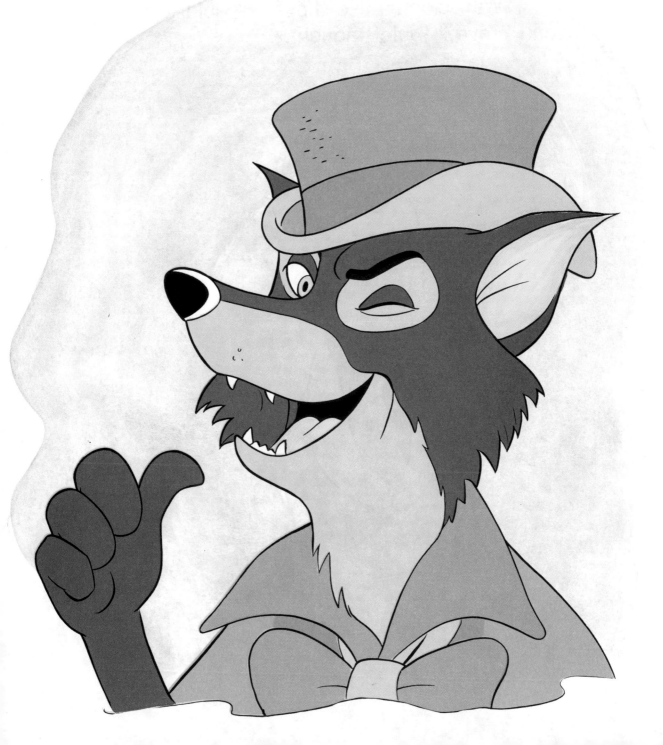

All the animals nodded and agreed. You could tell just by his clothes that Sly Fox was important.

"With clothes like those, I could look big and brave," Piglet thought.

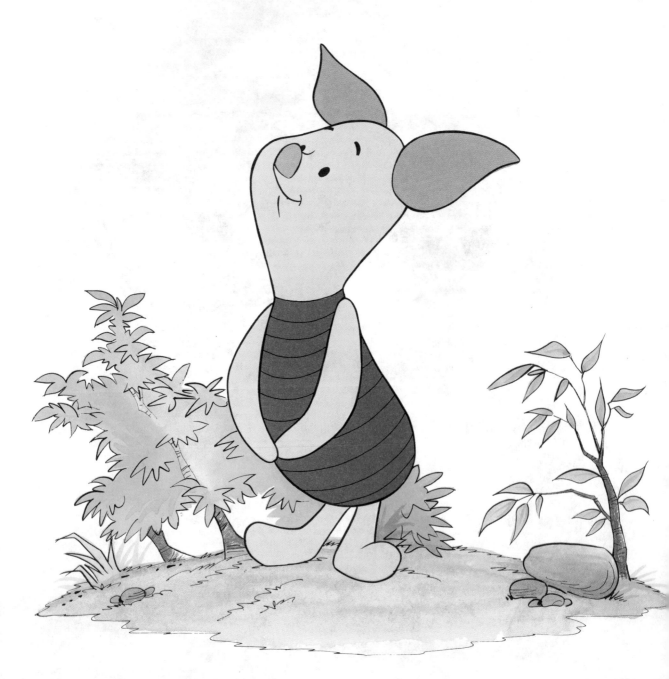

"Why, I could be the life of every party," thought Owl.

"They would make me feel almost happy," thought Eeyore.

"Where can I get some?" asked Tigger.

"Oh, do tell us, please," cried Kanga.

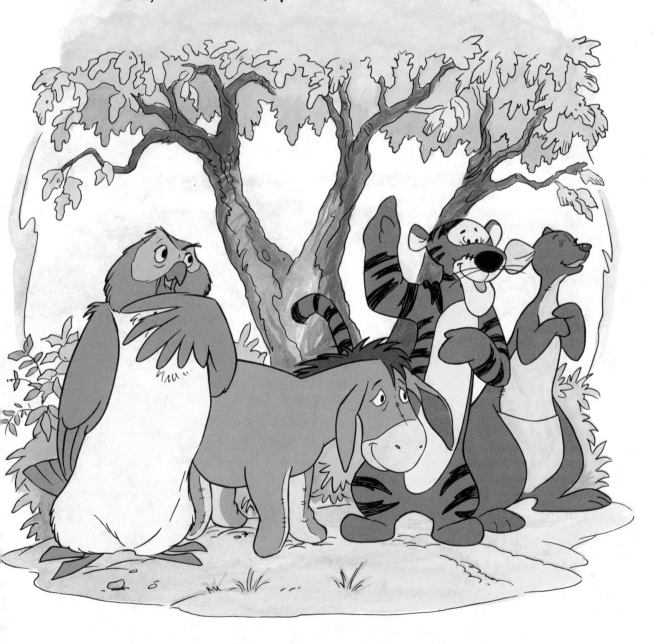

"I can make these clothes for you," said Sly Fox. "I have some of the best cloth ever made. No other cloth is as soft, as smooth, or as light. It is also magic cloth. Only <u>wise</u> people can see it."

"My word," muttered Owl.

"How wonderful," said Rabbit.

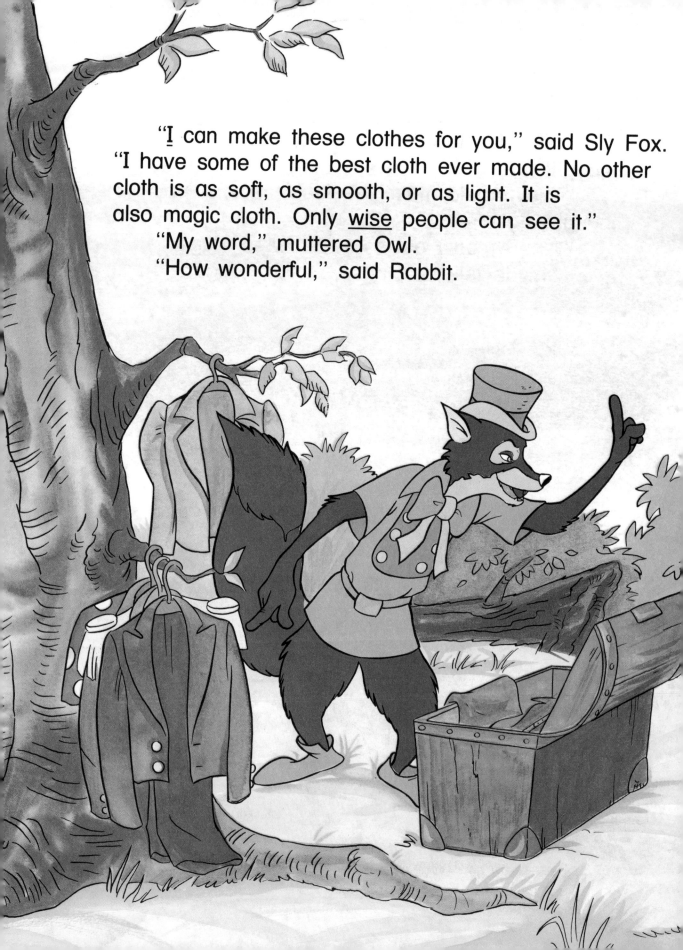

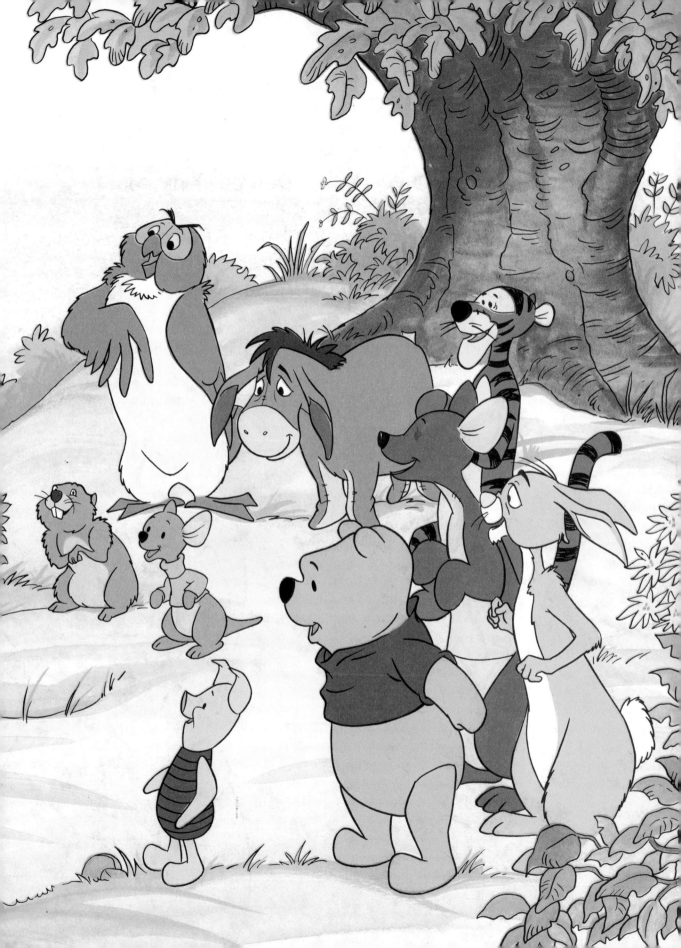

"Who will be the first to have clothes of magic cloth?" asked Sly.

"I will!" cried Pooh. "Do you think you could make a suit to fit me?"

"For a price, my good bear. For a price," said Sly, "I will make you a suit. But you must give me all of your honey."

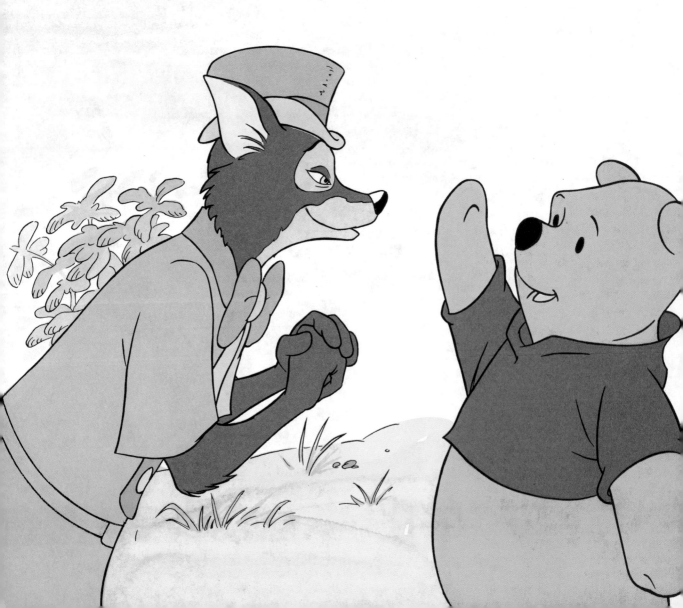

"Hmm," thought Pooh. "That is quite a lot to ask."

"Wear it, and you will be the wisest bear around," said Sly.

"Oh, all right," sighed Pooh.

"It is a deal," cried Sly.

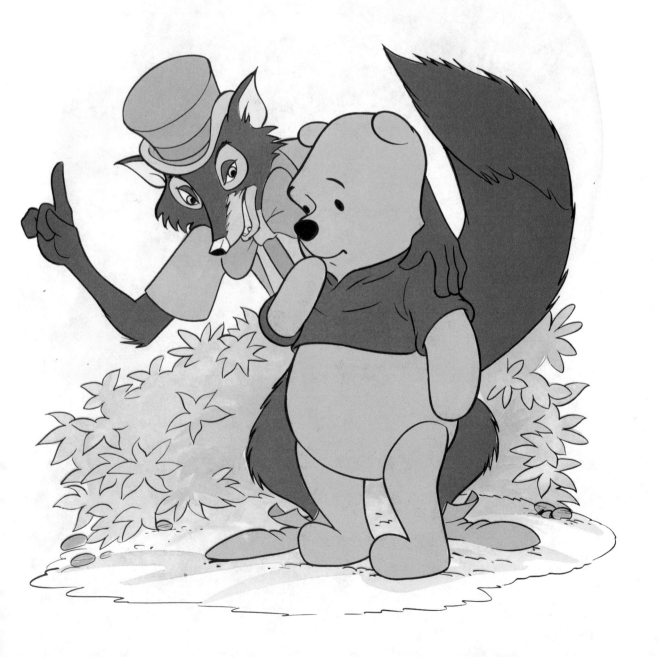

Sly Fox set up his shop in a quiet corner of the Wood. All the animals left him alone so that he could make Pooh's new clothes.

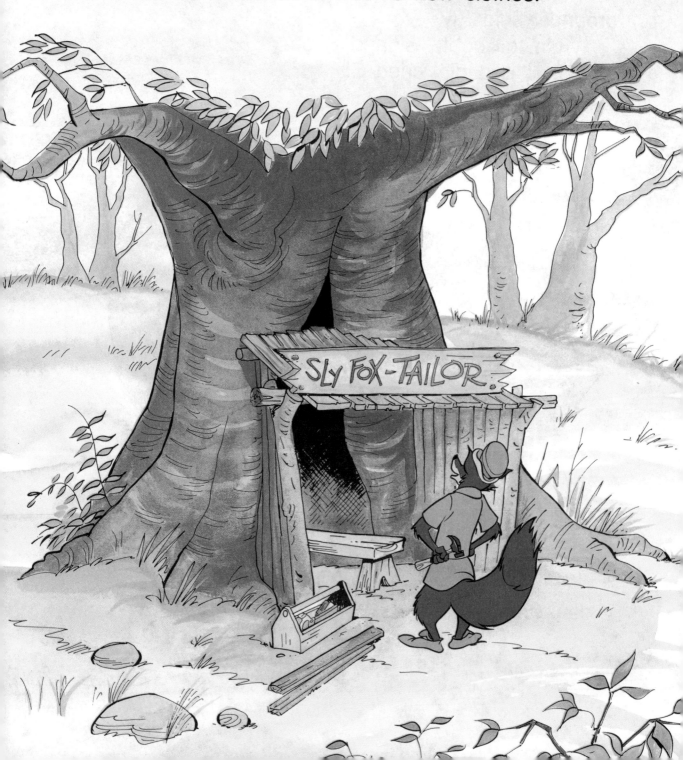

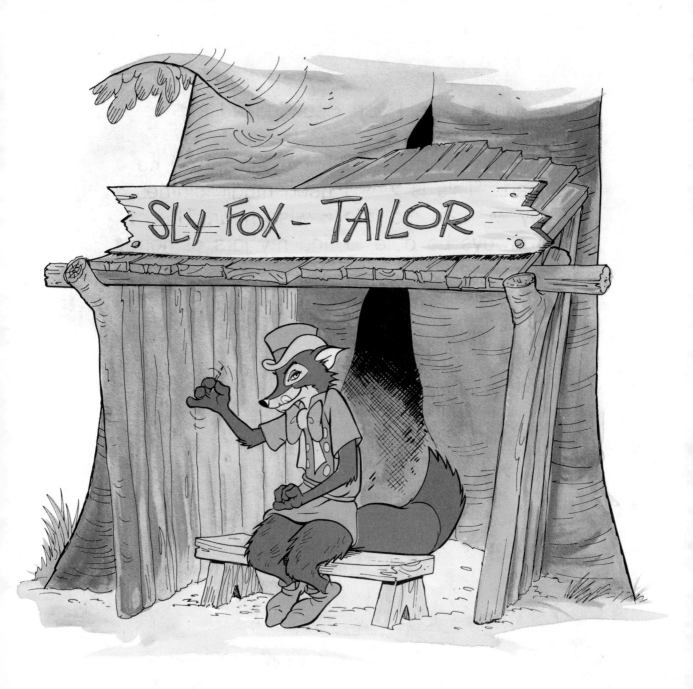

But Sly had played a trick on the good animals in the Hundred Acre Wood. There was no magic cloth at all! Day after day, Sly pretended to work. But all he really did was think about Pooh's delicious honey.

Meanwhile, Pooh Bear looked for his honey.

"Now where did I put those jars?" he sighed. "This is why I need magic clothes. <u>They</u> will turn me into a wise bear. Then I will always be able to find my jars of honey."

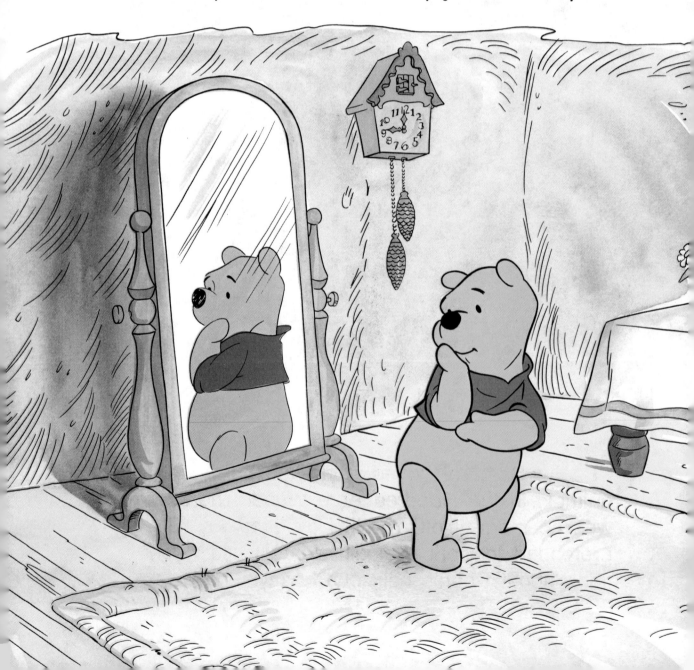

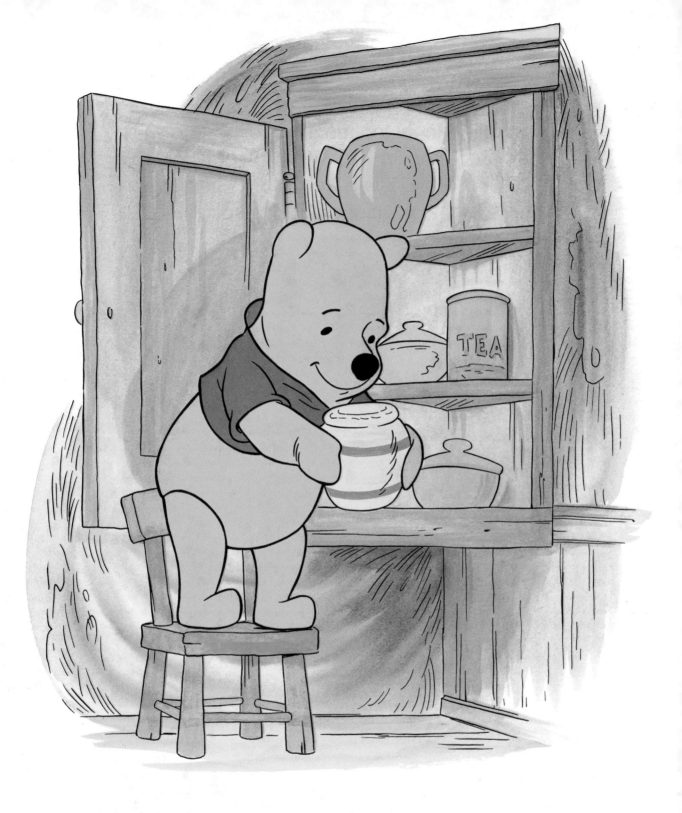

This thought pleased Pooh a lot. Now he
did not mind looking for the honey at all.

While Pooh looked for his honey, the
other creatures in the Wood began to worry.
"I do hope I will be able to see the
clothes of magic cloth," Piglet said.

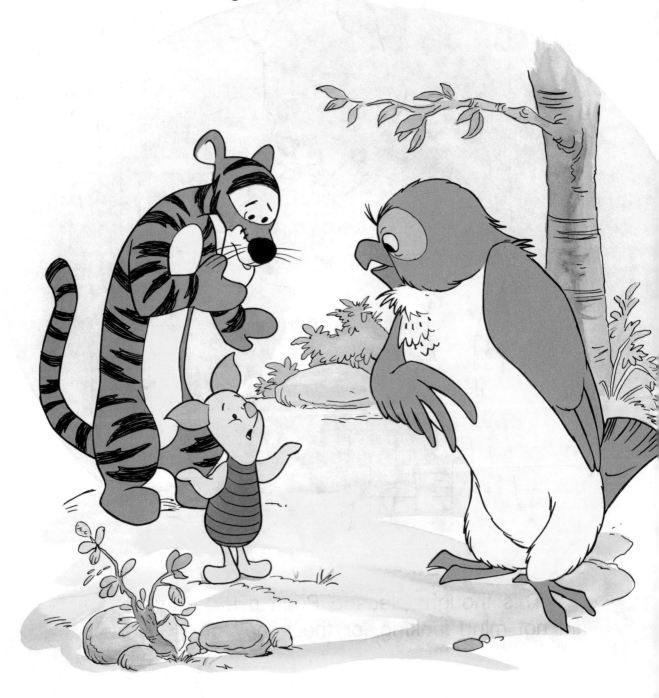

"Only wise people can see the clothes," said Owl. "I am sure that I will be able to see them."

"I know I will see them too," said Tigger. But he secretly wondered if he was wise enough.

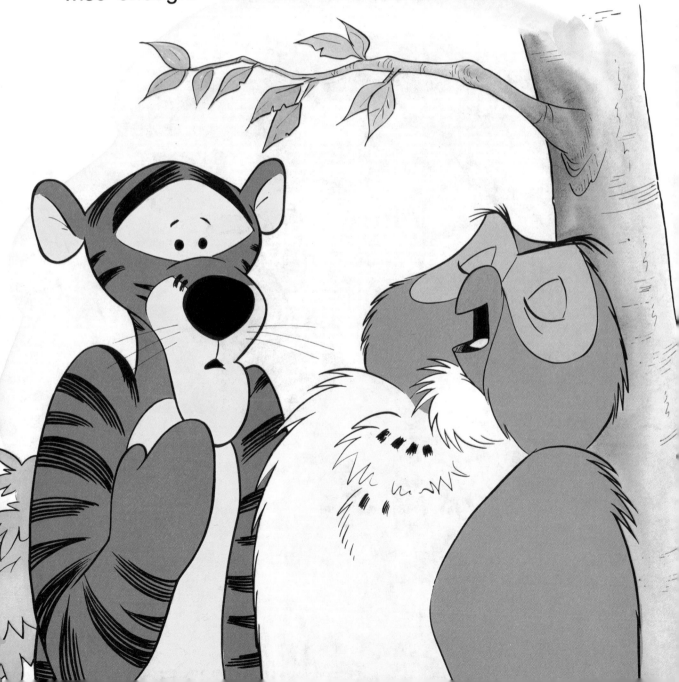

"Maybe none of us is wise enough to see the magic cloth," thought Tigger. He was worried.

"Well, I am off," he said. Then he bounced on over to Sly's workshop. He wanted to find out if he was wise or not.

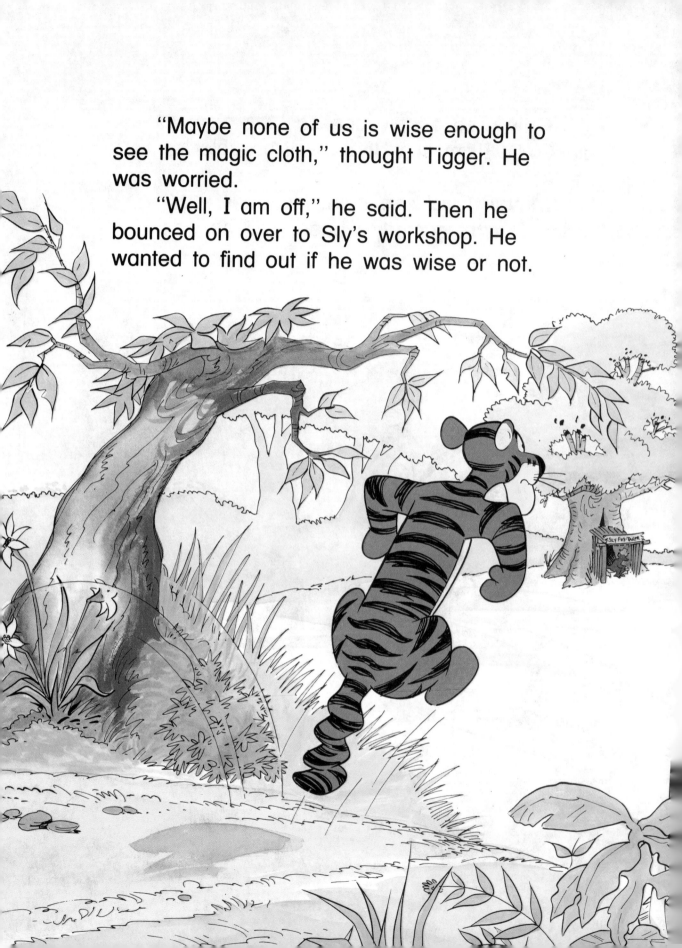

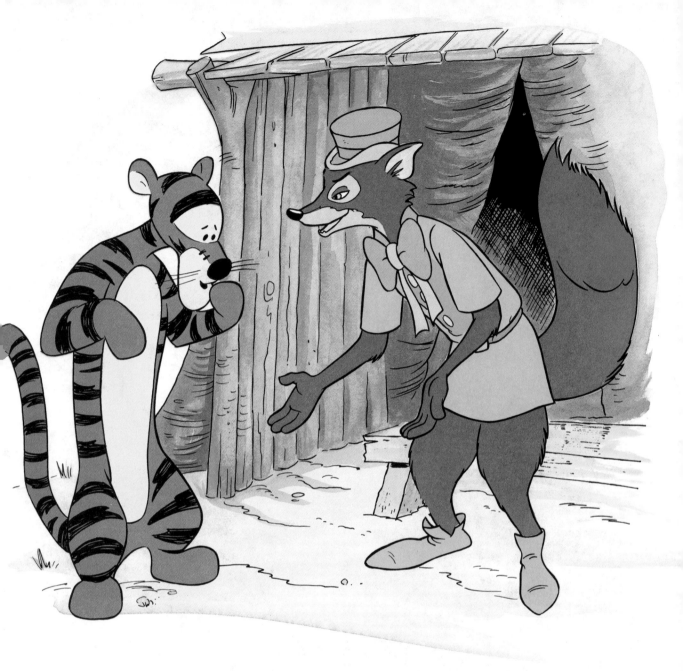

"Take a look," said Sly. "Isn't it lovely?"

"Uh-oh," thought Tigger. "I don't see anything at all!"

But that is not what Tigger said. He told Sly Fox it was the prettiest cloth he had ever seen. And he told the other animals the same thing.

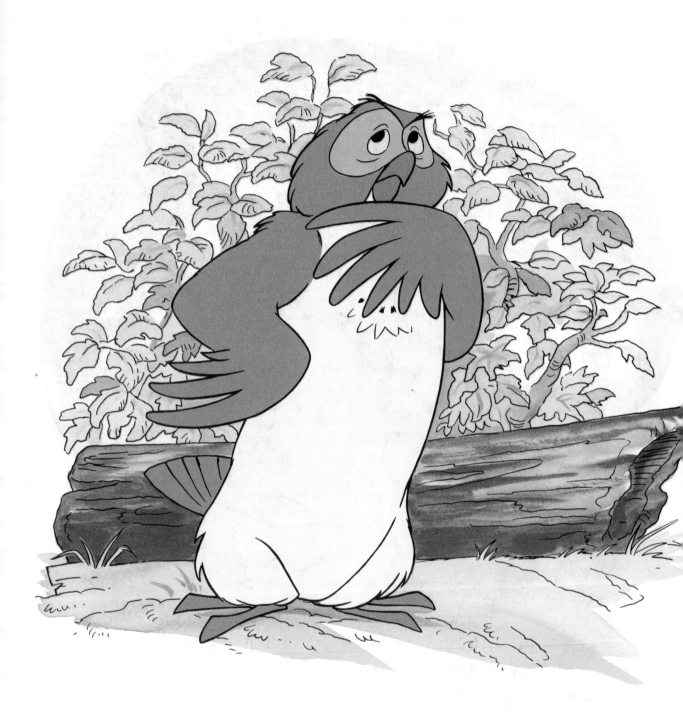

Soon Owl began to wonder if <u>he</u> was wise enough to see the magic cloth. He did not want to be the only one who could not see it. So Owl, too, went to visit Sly.

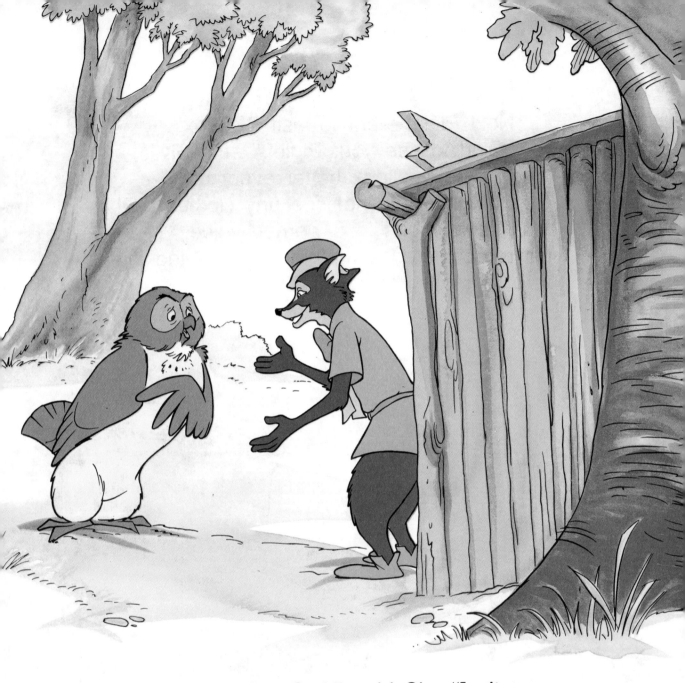

"See here, wise Owl," said Sly. "Isn't my cloth grand?"

Owl was about to say, "I don't see any cloth." But he remembered that even Tigger had seen it. "Yes, indeed. That cloth is grand." He walked away slowly, thinking very hard.

Next Piglet went to visit Sly Fox.

"Glad to see you, Piglet," said Sly.
"Pooh's clothes look better every day."

But Piglet did not see any clothes. "Oh,
dear," said Piglet in a worried voice. "I—I—
just remembered something—something I must
do at home!"

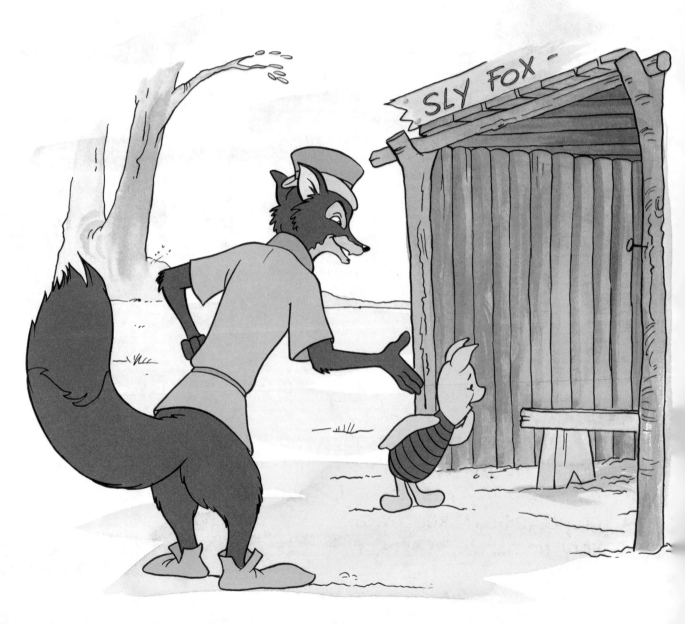

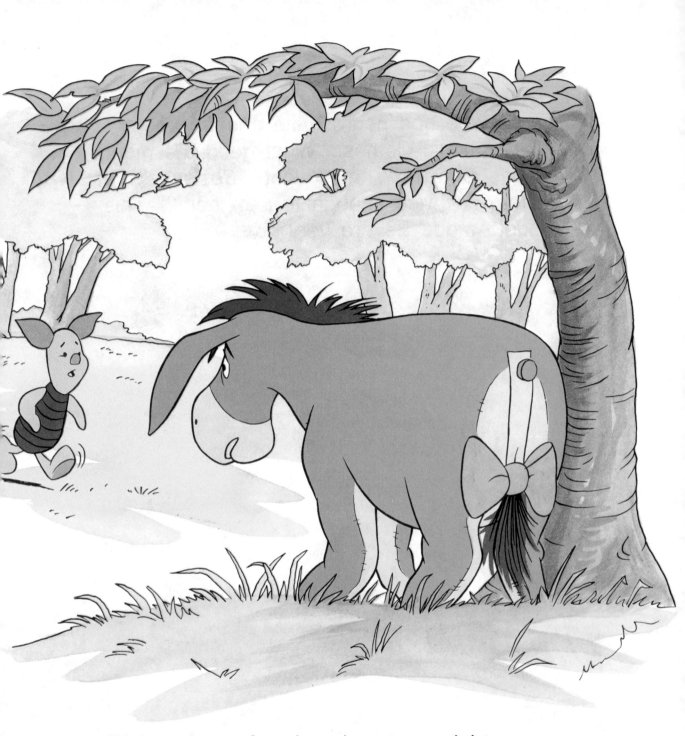

Piglet ran so fast he almost ran right
into Eeyore.

"Fine clothes," said Piglet nervously.
"Very fine clothes." He hurried away, shaking
his head.

Eeyore had heard quite enough about Pooh's magic clothes. "What good are magic clothes anyway?" he thought. "Besides, what if I am not wise enough to see them?" This thought made Eeyore very sad.

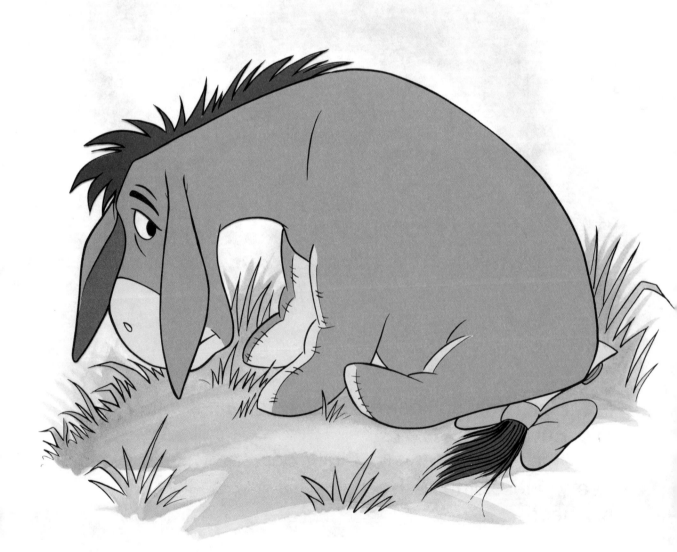

When he got to Sly's, Eeyore felt sadder than ever. "I <u>would</u> have to be the only one who cannot see Pooh's clothes!" he thought.

But Eeyore would not say that he could not see the clothes. So he muttered, "They are all right—if you like that kind of thing."

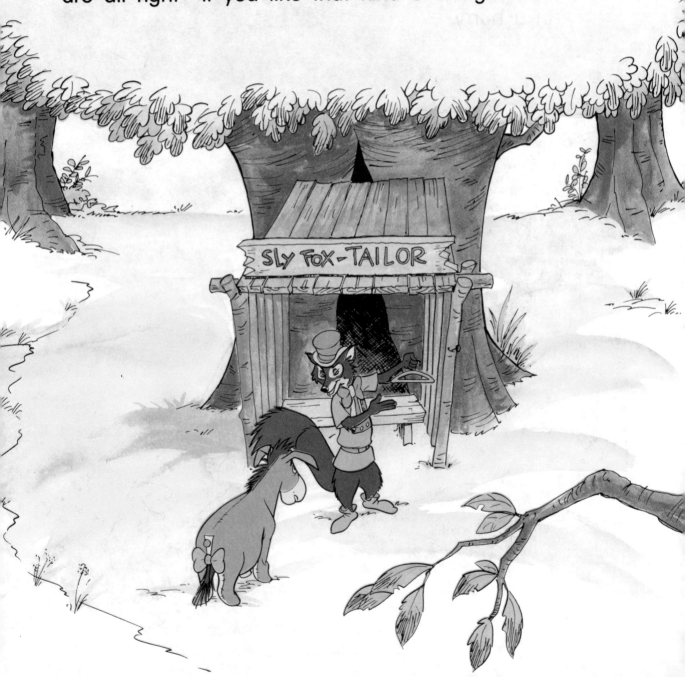

Kanga and Roo also went to visit Sly.

"Oh, Mr. Fox! How lovely," said Kanga.

"What is Mama making such a fuss about?" wondered Roo. "I don't see any—" Roo began to say.

"Hush, dear," said Kanga. Then she left in a hurry.

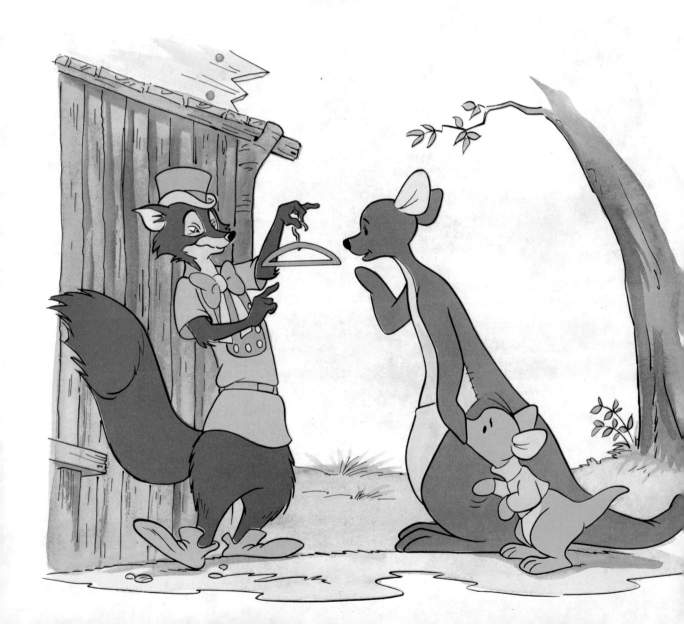

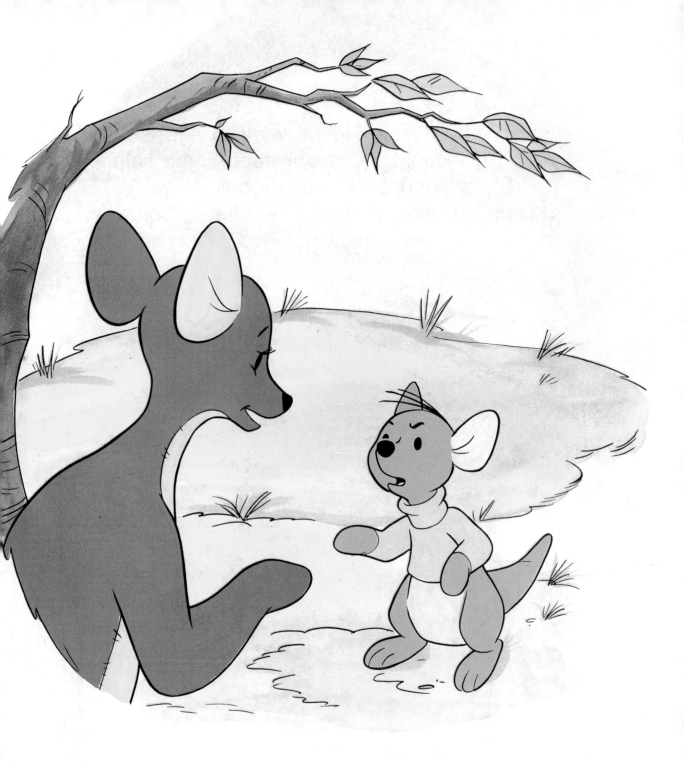

"But Mama, there were no clothes in Mr. Fox's shop!"

"I know that, dear," answered Kanga. "Just don't tell anyone else."

The next day, Rabbit went to see Sly Fox. He thought Sly might need some help. Sly was happy to see Rabbit. "The clothes are almost done," he cried. "Come inside and take a look!"

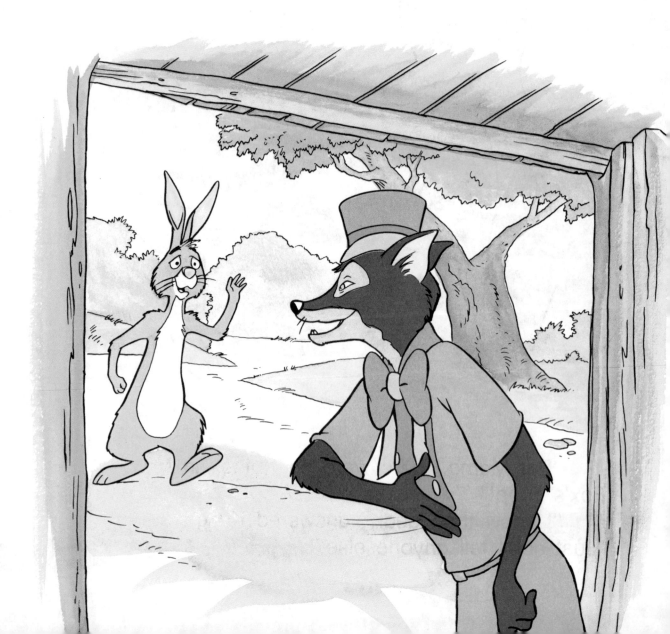

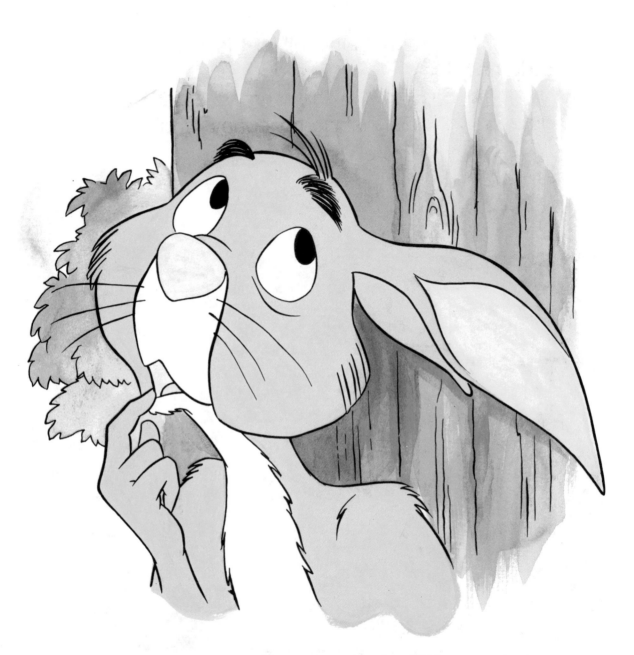

Rabbit stepped into the shop. "There
must be some mistake," he thought. "I do not
see a stitch of clothing anywhere."

But all Rabbit said was, "My, my! Those
clothes are wonderful, all right."

At last Pooh found all of his jars
of honey.
"Did Sly Fox say he wanted <u>all</u> of my
honey? Perhaps just <u>some</u> honey would do."

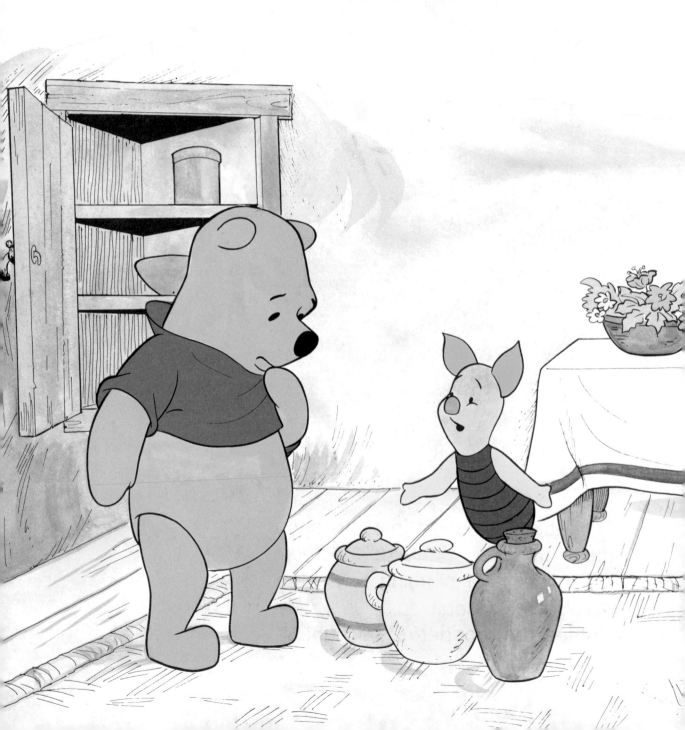

"He did say <u>all</u> your honey jars, Pooh. But think of what you will get," said Piglet.

"The best clothes in all the world," added Rabbit.

"Yes, you are right," sighed Pooh. He picked up all his honey jars. "Here I go!"

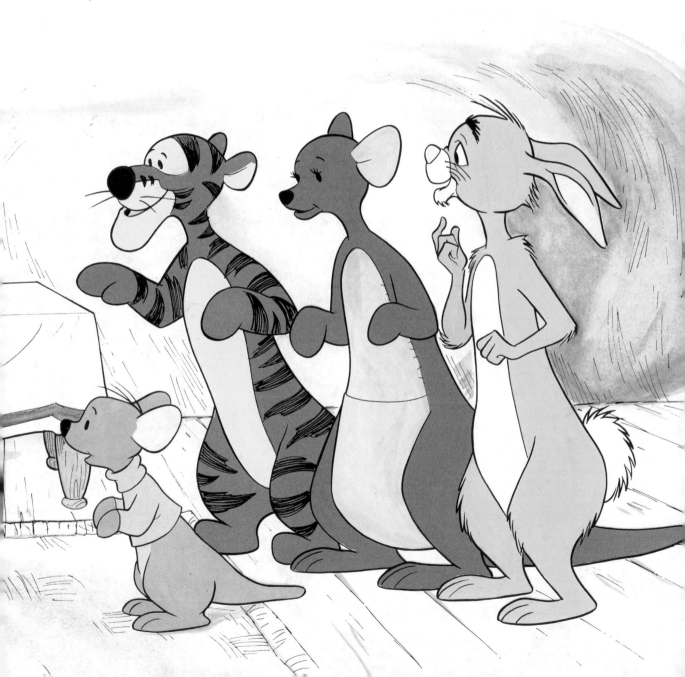

"Yum!" thought Sly when he saw Pooh's honey. He grabbed the jars. "Here is your grand new suit."

"Ooh!" said Tigger

"Aah!" said Rabbit.

"But . . ." said Roo.

"Hush!" said Kanga.

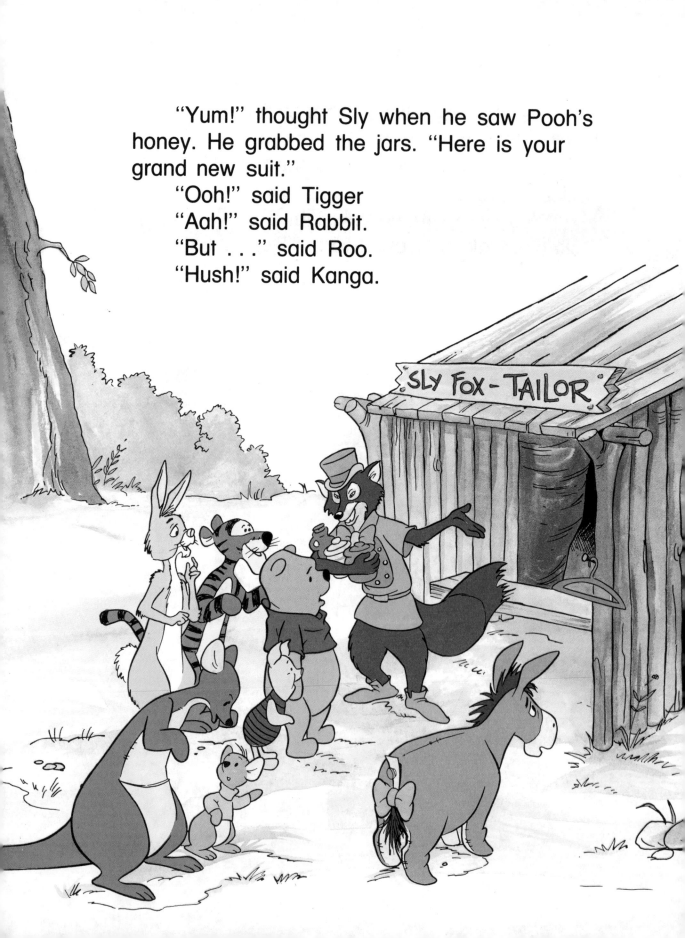

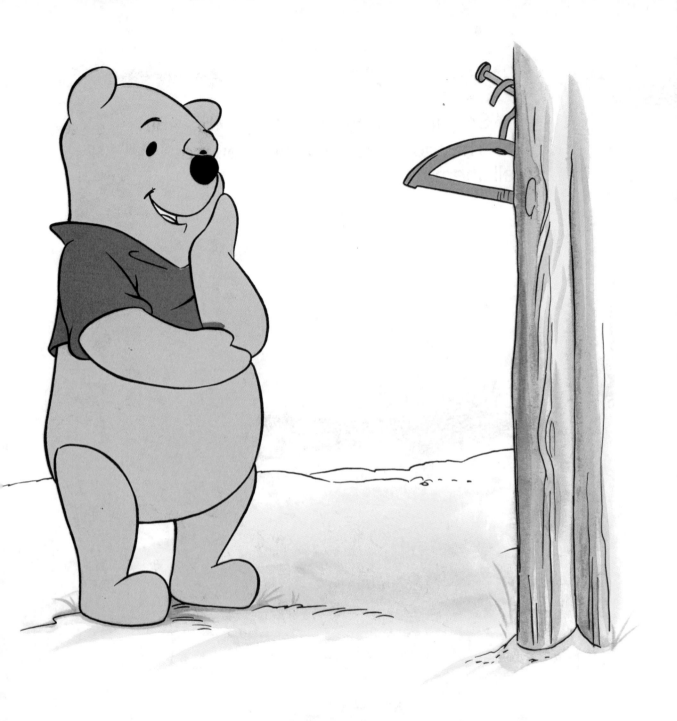

"I love them!" said Pooh. He did not care that <u>he</u> could not see the clothes. He knew he was just a bear of little brain. But Pooh was glad that his wise friends could see them. That was enough for him.

"See the pretty flowers on the shirt?" asked Sly. "They look so real that you can almost smell them."

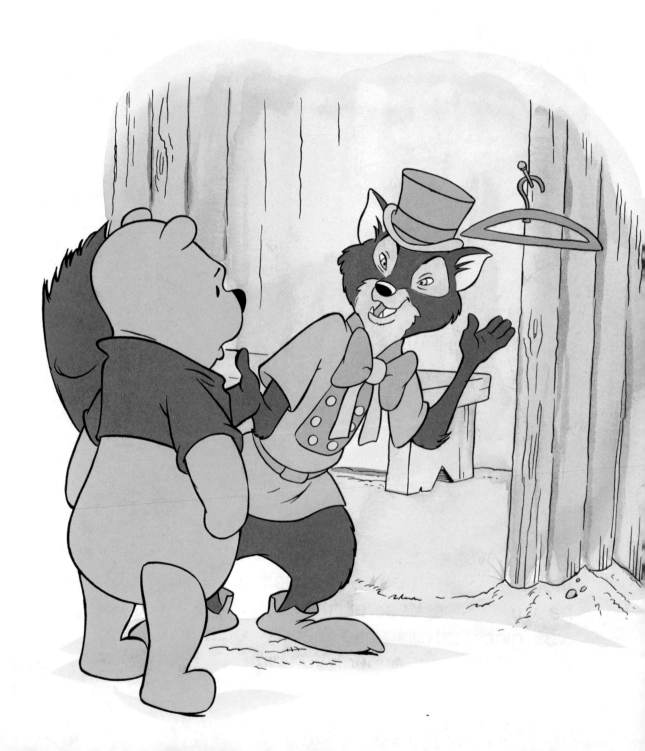

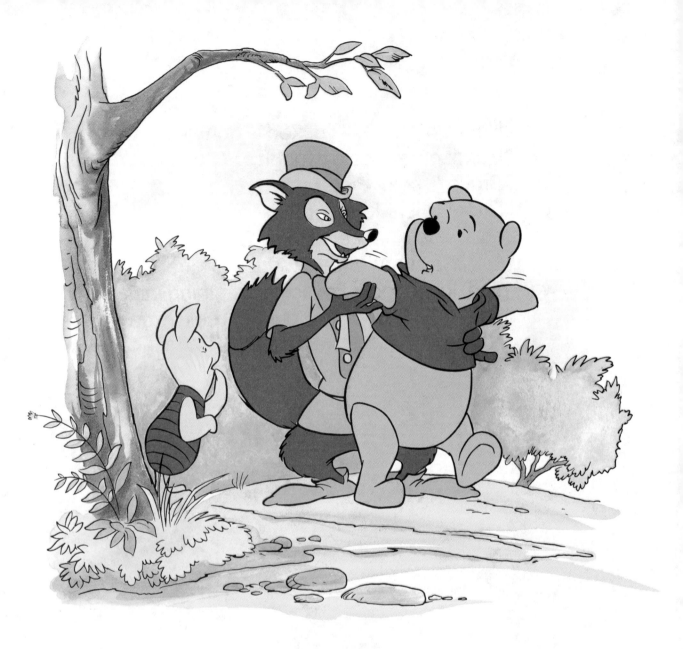

As Pooh sniffed the air, Sly pretended to help Pooh put on his new shirt and pants. "Pretty good fit, aren't they? Now for the jacket," said Sly. "A beautiful suit. And it is so light in weight that you won't even know you are wearing it!"

"That's true," said Pooh in a small voice.

"How do I look?" asked Pooh.
"Handsome," said Kanga.
"Brave," said Piglet.
"Happy," said Eeyore.
"Not wise?" asked Pooh Bear.
"Oh yes, very wise," added Tigger. He was glad to be able to say something nice.
"That's just what I thought," said Pooh.

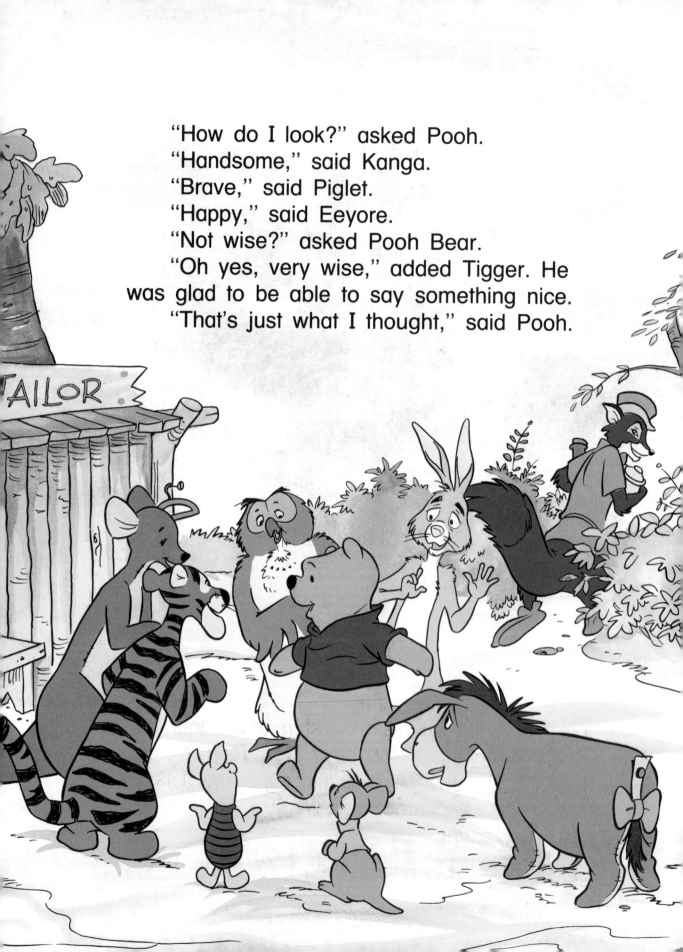

TAILOR

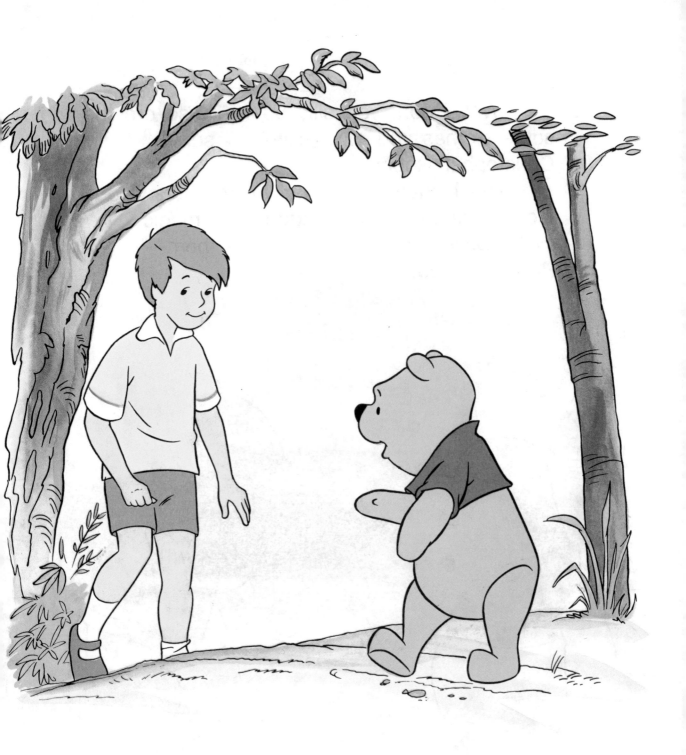

Just then Pooh saw Christopher Robin.
"What do you think of my new clothes,
Christopher Robin?" asked Pooh.

"Why Pooh, you silly bear. Those are the same clothes you always wear," said Christopher Robin.

"But I gave Sly Fox all of my honey to make these. They are made from magic cloth. Only wise people can see them—" Pooh stopped.

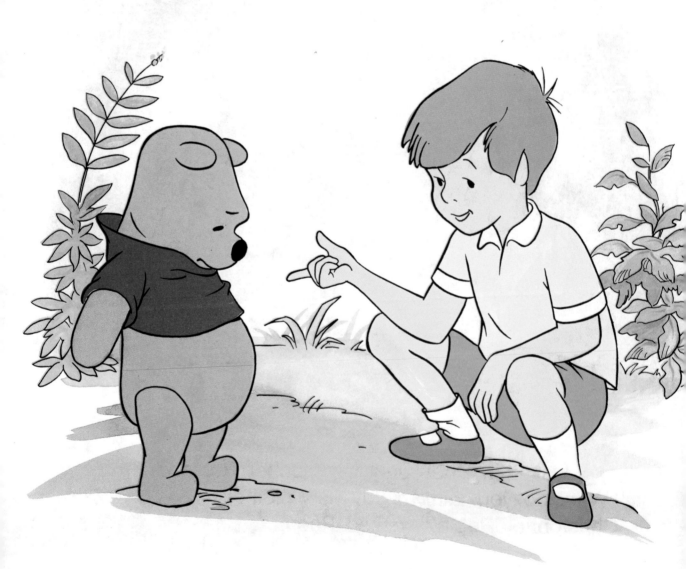

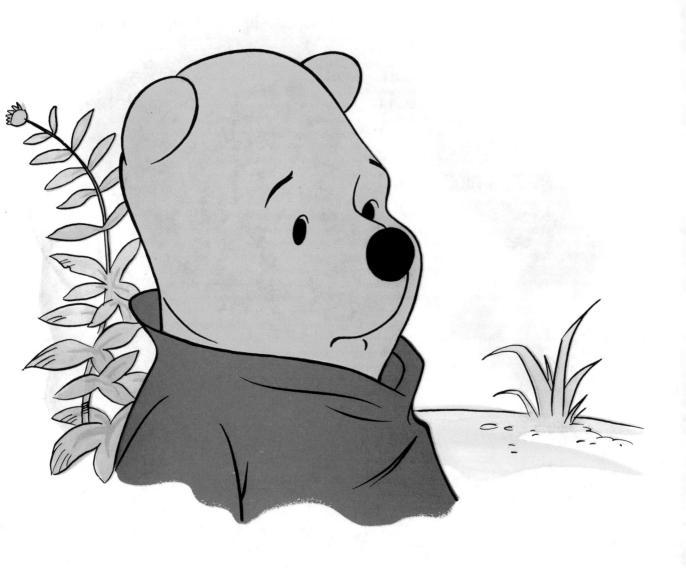

Suddenly Pooh Bear knew the truth.
There was no one wiser than Christopher
Robin. If he could not see the clothes, they
just were not there.

"That Sly Fox played a trick on me," he
said. "I wish I had kept a little honey. It helps
to have honey at a time like this."

"Don't feel bad, Pooh. Sly Fox tricked us all," said Owl.

"I knew there was no cloth," said Roo.

"All of you knew," said Christopher Robin, "but you were afraid to believe your own eyes. You were afraid of what the others would think. But I think you are all perfect just the way you are."

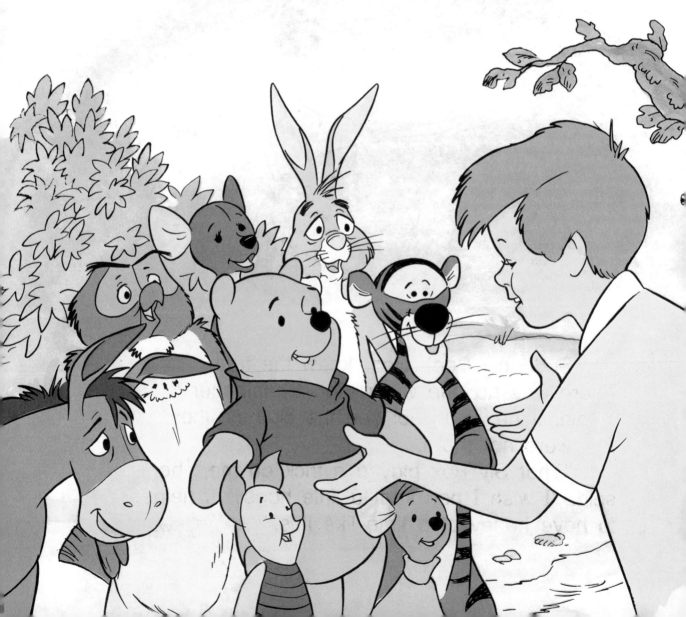

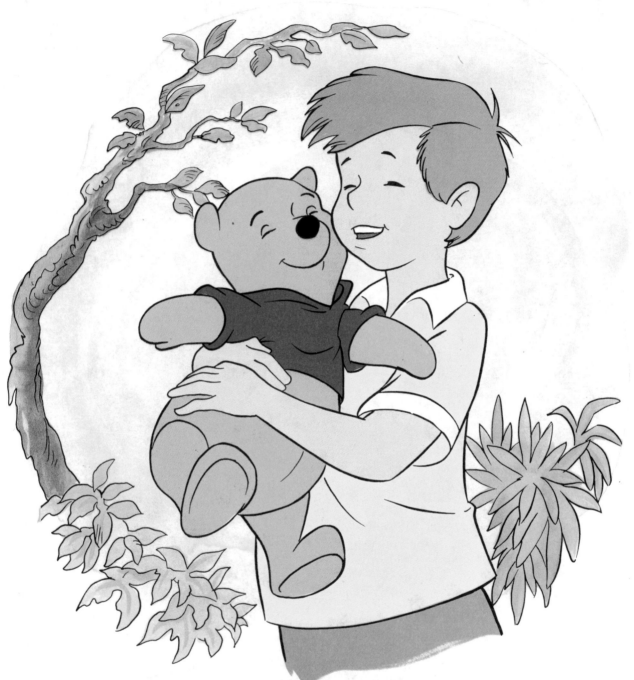

Then Christopher Robin took them home. And he gave Pooh Bear an extra hug to show him he was the best bear in the whole wide world.

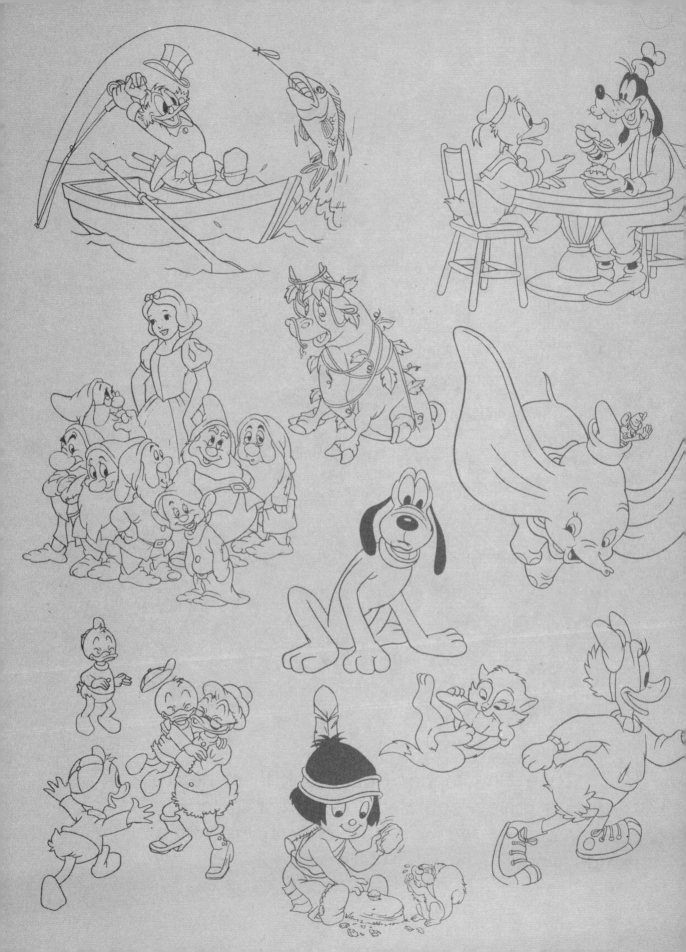